AROMATHERAPY: MY WAY

AROMATHERAPY: MY WAY

by

Marjorie Helliwell–Shakespeare

Pentland Books
Edinburgh · Durham · Oxford

© Marjorie Helliwell-Shakespeare 2001

First published in 2001 by
Pentland Books
1 Hutton Close
South Church
Bishop Auckland
Durham

British Library Cataloguing in Publication Data.
A catalogue record for this book is available
from the British Library.

ISBN 1 85821 916 7

Typeset by George Wishart & Associates, Whitley Bay.
Printed and bound by Antony Rowe Ltd., Chippenham.

CONTENTS

THE HISTORY OF MASSAGE

For as long as man can remember, massage has been practised all over the world in one form or another. In the most ancient writings it records the beneficial effects.

It appears that massage was used as a remedial agent long before medicine or any other allied science was understood.

Massage is a scientific manipulation of soft tissues for healing purposes, and the object of massage is the restoration of normal function.

Of all the arts, massage is one of the most respected, but its application depends entirely on the personal skill of the therapist's hands.

The earliest known references to massage are contained in Kong-Fu's Chinese White Books, which are of unknown antiquity, but probably written about 3000BC. It is also mentioned in the Sacred Books of the Hindus, besides the very earliest historical accounts of the Egyptians, Greeks, Persians and Romans.

The Greeks, in particular, developed a well arranged system of massage and even Homer in 1000BC refers to the benefits of massage in his famous Odyssey. He infers that the most beautiful of women rubbed their heroes with aromatic oils and were able to ease the fatigue of exhausted warriors.

In 500BC Herodicus, who was a most learned Greek physician, insisted that all his patients were 'to be rubbed thoroughly', and from this period there followed the appointment of gymnasia throughout the whole of Greece.

Two of the most ancient and greatest philosophers, Socrates and Plato, made some of their famous discourses during their restorative treatments at the beautifully designed and appointed gymnasia.

Hippocrates, 460BC, also known as the Father of Medicine, in his writings on the use of medicinal herbs, was more specific in his use of massage and made some definite scientific deductions. He made the first broad classification of movements and on one occasion, whilst speaking of rubbing, pointed out that things 'which have the same name do not always have the same effect.'

Hippocrates stated that 'rubbing can bind a joint that is too loose and loosen a joint that is too tight. Massage can bind or loosen, it can both make flesh, and yet cause flesh to waste. Hard rubbing binds, soft rubbing loosens, much rubbing causes parts to waste. Slight or soft rubbing makes parts grow.'

Hippocrates made many useful observations. He recommended friction for sprains and abdominal massage for constipation. He appreciated the value of massage or 'rubbing' in acute paralysis, rheumatism and obesity. Although he did not understand the circulatory system, which was not understood for approximately another 2000 years, he was careful and observant enough to see that rubbing an extremity upwards was more productive than rubbing downwards.

In general, we may say that his findings are still consistent with modern day teaching and, of course, medical graduates still take the Hippocratic Oath.

Eventually the Romans absorbed a great deal of the Grecian culture. Asclepiades, a Greek, was practising a type of physiotherapy in Rome, shortly before the birth of Christ.

Julius Caesar, 55BC, suffered from epilepsy and used to be pinched all over as a counter irritant to the neuralgic pains he had.

Headaches were also relieved by 'rubbing' and flaccid paralysis was helped by massage.

One of the great pioneers in medicine was Galen, 130 AD. He was responsible for the first catalogue of medicinal plants. He took a considerable interest in the possibilities of physical treatment. Prior to his discovery that blood was in the arteries, it had always been assumed that these vessels contained air, hence the name. He had plenty of opportunity to study the circulatory system as he was appointed physician to the Roman gladiators! He also instituted a preparatory 'rubbing' for the champions whose bodies were slapped until they were red and then smeared them with aromatic oils.

This type of massage or rubbing continued into the Middle Ages, when, like many other arts, it fell into disuse until 1584, when the outstanding French surgeon, Ambrose Pare, vigorously revived the art.

His infinite care of all his surgical cases made him most selective in his choice of movements and his explicit instructions are still preserved to this day.

About this time in history, massage and remedial exercises progressed in England by Timothy Bright; in Germany by Leonard Fuchs and in Italy by Hieronymus Mercurials. Each of these men wrote very valuable material on these subjects.

Lord Bacon said that rubbing or friction made the parts more fleshy and full. He wrote, 'the cause is that they draw a greater quantity of blood to the parts, they draw the ailments more forcibly from within, they relax the pores and make a better passage or escape for the spirit, blood or ailment, and lastly they dissipate and digest moisture which lieth in the flesh, all which helps assimilation'.

The King of Prussia was given rubbings by Hoffman in 1706 and massage was practised about this time in many parts of the Continent, although no exact system had yet been established. Famous physicians and surgeons once again began to use massage in the treatment of injuries and disease.

Massage was the main terminology used, but new words such as pressure, kneading and manipulation were introduced.

In Oxford in 1800 a well known surgeon, Grosvenor, cured stiff joints by physical methods, and soon afterwards, Balfour of Edinburgh became famous for similar treatment.

Probably the greatest name associated with massage was Peter Ling (1776-1839). He was a Swede who, in 1813, founded the Gymnastic Central Institute at Stockholm, which even today remains the foremost teaching school in the world. Ling was a teacher of fencing and gymnastics, and not only did he start a new massage system, but he correlated all the work of past and contemporary gymnasts, and placed the study of the subject onto a scientific basis. He classified all gymnastic movements into either passive, active, or resisted. He rated massage as a passive movement.

He founded the Swedish system of massage and exercise and introduced terms such as 'effleurage', 'petrissage', 'vibration' and 'friction' as well as 'rolling', 'slapping', 'pinching' and other descriptions of massage.

However, despite the good work and promotion of massage by Peter Ling, it was not until the end of the 19th century that massage began to be favoured and accepted all over the world as an orthodox method of treatment. Previous to this, training was inadequate and women engaged in massage were generally of ill repute and opportunists and this flourished during the First World War.

After this it became necessary to obtain a special licence in the London area before the practice of massage was permitted. To become a student of massage it was necessary for a British student to travel to Stockholm to study this science. In 1894 a small group of educated women formed the first Society of Trained Masseuses and, in 1900, they became Incorporated.

After 1919 women students were admitted for training and in 1920 the Incorporated Society was granted a Royal Charter, which later became known as the Chartered Society of Massage and Remedial Exercise. The title was changed again in 1943 to the Chartered Society of Physiotherapy. State Registration came in 1964. Massage at last was given the stamp of respectability by the medical profession and the State for the treatment of disease and injury.

However, there was still an urgent need to raise the standards of massage of practitioners in the beauty field, so the London Institute looked into the possibility of providing further education and training for girls wishing to study beauty massage and in establishing a nationally recognized course.

In 1970 the first City and Guilds Beauty Therapy examination took place. There are now several other associations, private schools and colleges in the British Isles and each one has different motives and aims. But, the ultimate objective is the same – to gain a recognized professional diploma.

THE THEORY OF MASSAGE

❧

Every profession calls for courage and determination and this is no exception. No training school can make you successful. It can teach you technique and it can indicate the ways towards a successful practice and career.

A therapist must try to first equip themselves with knowledge, study and practise all movements.

They must try to cultivate a quiet, confident and professional manner and aim for the highest ideals. They must give care for every client or patient, irrespective of age, sex or status.

The therapist must learn to manipulate soft tissue with reverence, for the body is the most wonderful creation in the world.

The body is composed of living cells eager to respond to stimulation.

These tissues experience all the many sensations that vary from exquisite pleasure to acute pain. The soft, resilient and relaxed muscle will obediently remain passive to hands that can mould their way into its midst, but presents a hard, contracted and suspicious mass to the digital assault of inquisitive prods.

Muscles respond to consideration and understanding. Therefore, hands must be trained.

Well trained hands can stimulate the nutrition to the area by bringing more blood to the area and by causing an interchange of fluids within the tissues. They can remove and prevent the formation of adhesive, soft, scar tissue; remove swelling and promote the disposal of congestion. Some movements can help stimulate the nerves, while others soothe them.

Other movements can help in paralysis and ease the pain of sciatica, neuritis, neuralgia and similar conditions and can be efficacious in respiratory and abdominal diseases.

Often massage techniques will produce amazing results when all other treatments have failed, as it is a powerful therapeutic agent.

Massage consists essentially of movements performed on a passive patient and complete relaxation is, therefore, of the greatest importance. Relaxation and comfort are almost synonymous and the first aim of the therapist should always be to obtain the most comfortable position for the patient, consistent with accessibility of the parts. Relaxed tissues greatly facilitate good massage.

The question of lubricants in massage is usually a personal preference. It is permissible to use a non-starchy, unscented, finely sifted talcum powder. It should never be applied directly to the patient but, instead, dusted on the therapist's hands. The same rule applies to oils and other lubricants.

The use of powder permits a smooth slide on the body and is ideal for a general body massage.

Whenever there is a hair growth, it is better to use a fine cream or aromatic oil, which is also more suitable for abdominal massage when the abdomen is hard and contracted.

Oils should always be used on dry, mature skin as this assists in the removal of dry, hard and flaked skin accumulation. This applies over scar tissue, as this helps to nourish the weakened tissues. Many medicaments are used in various creams and oils, but their efficacy depends on the skill of the therapist.

The physiological effects of massage are just as important. Special movements in massage provoke effects both physiologically and pathologically. In today's practice the aim of massage is to restore normal function.

The human body is simply a mass of living cells, each dependent upon the assimilation of certain food products for its activity.

Activation, or heat and energy, is brought about by oxidation. Food products and oxygen are carried to the cells by lymph.

Health, movement and repair depends entirely upon renewed and continual interchange of lymph within the tissues. If this can be established and maintained, healing and physiological recovery will normally take place. Thus the foundation of massage theory:

THE EFFECTS UPON THE CIRCULATION
Massage speeds up the blood flow.

Effleurage encourages the venous return and lymphatic flow. The presence of valves in the vessels makes sure that blood and lymph can only flow in one direction, that is towards the heart. Massage can mechanically empty these vessels and, since a vacuum cannot exist in the body, they are immediately refilled, and in this way the venous system is materially assisted.

Petrissage movement causes a temporary difference in the shape of a muscle. This produces a direct pumping effect and causes an acceleration in the blood flow. It also assists cardiac action, without increasing the work of the heart. It increases the number of red and white corpuscles in the blood and raises the haemoglobin content by 25%. Massage does not assist in their formation, but brings them into the blood stream, therefore giving the patient a feeling of well-being.

THE EFFECTS ON THE DIGESTIVE SYSTEM
These functions are dependent upon the lymph and blood supply.

The arterial blood is increased, the secretion of digestive juices become more prolific, and the portal and hepatic systems are increased in function. Massage to the abdomen helps normal digestion, absorption and excretion. It also produces more red corpuscles and helps pass food products more quickly into the system. It also slightly increases the blood pressure.

THE EFFECTS UPON METABOLISM

Metabolism is the process of life by which tissue cells are destroyed by combustion and renewed from chemical substances carried by the blood derived from digested foods. Massage increases the metabolic rate. It benefits carbohydrate and fat metabolism, decreases the blood pressure, increases the quantity of urine and temperature by promotion of heat. These are three very important curative factors.

THE EFFECTS ON THE MUSCULAR SYSTEM

The effects of massage on the muscular system are very marked. Massage cannot, and does not, increase the size of a muscle, but it does, and can, maintain its tone, free it from waste products that hinder its function, and restore it to normal activity.

The shape, the contour and beauty depends upon the tone of the skeletal muscles. It is an entirely muscular compression which squeezes along the lymph and blood in the veins. The muscular system controls respiration and many other vital organs.

Life is movement and all movement is a process of combustive oxidation, which produces an ash. This is usually acid and can be either butyric, lactic, carbonic or uric. All these are normal products, but when they exist together in the body they become fatigue products. Their presence is the direct cause of fatigue. In small amounts these irritants are easily removed by the lymphatic glands, but if they are in excess they produce swelling, aching and muscular rheumatism.

Exercise will develop a muscle. At the same time, fatigue products increase, which massage will break down and eliminate by encouraging the flow into the lymphatic system. Massage will improve the blood supply to the muscles to nourish and prevent the formation of irritants. It counteracts the wastage of disuse. Massage will produce local heat and imparts tone to the muscle cells.

THE EFFECTS UPON THE NERVOUS SYSTEM

The nervous system is so allied to the muscular system that it is often referred to as the neuro-muscular system. Strong and continued pressure with massage lessens the conductivity of a nerve, whereas a light pressure stimulates it. Deep local pressure will relieve spasm or cramp and a rapid hacking excites normal reflexes.

Stimulation may be exerted upon all sensory nerve endings and this can be produced over the entire cerebro-spinal system. The increased blood supply, which all nerve endings receive, renews activity.

Light and gentle massage stimulates the general nervous system. A heavy massage produces a deadening effect. Indirectly, the secretory nerves are also stimulated.

THE EFFECTS ON THE SKIN

The skin is an extremely sensitive organ and responds to almost any stimulation. It covers the whole body and weighs approximately three kilograms for a person weighing 75 kilograms. It contains blood vessels, millions of cells, hairs, nerve endings, oil glands, sweat glands and sensory cells.

Massage brings about an increase in blood supply, which in turn nourishes and tones the tissues. It will remove dead cells of the corium and any other excretory or foreign products which prevent normal function. It soothes and excites cutaneous nerves according to the degree of pressure. It increases glandular function, both sebaceous and sudorific.

THE EFFECTS ON OTHER SYSTEMS

As lymph is in communication with every tissue of the body, general massage gives a feeling of fitness and well-being.

The respiratory system, largely governed by muscles, is benefited.

The pleurae and pleural cavities are nourished.

Nourishment is given to the synovial membranes of all moveable joints in the body.

Massage influences the growth of bone because its existence depends upon a full blood supply.

THE PRACTICE OF MASSAGE

❧

As always, massage must be accurately applied. In today's teaching, massage manipulations are divided into four principal headings.

1. **Effleurage** – a soothing, stroking movement, which may be performed in several different ways:
   a. stroking with the palm of one hand, or both hands
   b. stroking with the ball of the thumb
   c. stroking with the tips of the fingers
   The movement with the palm of the hand should be used on the extremities, and the neck.
   Both hands should be used on the trunk, particularly the back.
   Effleurage with the thumbs is used on small muscles, such as the face, hands or feet, and muscles that require individual attention.
   Fingertip effleurage is used with all facial massage, around joints, and for treatment of the fingers and toes. The pressure applied with this treatment varies from the slightest touch, to very vigorous squeezing.
   Effleurage movements should always be given upwards, that is towards the heart. When treating the upper extremity, the movements should be from the hand to the axilla, and on the lower extremity, from the toes to the groin.
   The stroking movement is ideal for painful conditions. Given lightly and smoothly, it tends to eradicate pain. Moderately heavy, it empties the veins and lymphatics, relieving oedema, swellings and products of inflammation.

2. **Frictions** – a movement performed either by using thumbs or finger tips.

The friction movements are performed quite forcibly, by pressing on to the underlying tissues, moving the skin with it.

The aim of friction movements is to loosen hardened tissue around tendons, ligaments and joints. Also where deposits, the result of inflammation, are causing pain.

Moderate to heavy pressure is used to crush and reduce conditions, so that they may be carried away in the circulation.

Frictions are used on flat muscles, such as the erector spinae. It is an excellent movement for the condition fibrositis.

3. **Petrissage** – also known as kneading, pinching, plucking or rolling. This movement is used for the lifting of muscles:
   a. with one hand
   b. with fingers and thumbs
   c. with both hands

The hands can be used in many ways, according to the area undergoing treatment.

The muscle should be treated like a sponge that requires squeezing out. It should be grasped by the entire bulk, lifting it free from its underlying tissue. Care must be taken not to pinch.

Individual muscles are picked out and kneaded. The circulation is stimulated, and petrissage is very valuable in the treatment of muscle strain.

The scalp may be treated by kneading or pinching or plucking with the fingers and thumbs.

Facial muscles may be rolled between fingers and thumbs, as in a beauty massage.

4. **Tapotément or Percussion** – movements are given to shake the tissues. The following movements also come under this heading:
   a. **hacking** – this is performed with the straight ulnar side of hands, moving the hands very rapidly, like a scissor movement.

b. **cupping** – is performed by forming a hollow cup with the hand, and striking the muscles very rapidly. The cushion of air prevents pain or bruising to the client. This movement is also known as clapping or boating.

c. **shaking** – the extremity of a limb, hand or foot is held firmly in both hands, and is freely and rapidly shaken.

d. **beating** – this is done with the fists lightly clenched. The muscles are then beaten rapidly. This beating movement must take place from the wrist, not from the elbow or shoulder.

e. **digital vibration** – a very difficult movement to acquire. Used mainly on motor points. The three middle fingers, or sometimes only one, are placed in position on the skin, the hand is then rapidly vibrated, moving the tissues with it.

Tapotément movements result in an increase in blood supply, a lessening of nerve irritability, and an increase in the contractability of muscle tissue.

All massage movements are put together to form a pattern, and general body or facial treatments are produced. Each massage could differ slightly, depending on the client's requirements.

If applied correctly the body should glow, with a feeling of well-being. This marvellous tonic effect is not only confined to the normal healthy person, but its value has now been recognized by psychiatrists, doctors and, particularly, the beauty care profession.

Physical and mental health is the basis of beauty, and in the busy, average day when all systems are go, tensions mount and relaxation is impossible.

These tensions of the mind and body begin to show on the face and in the body, which ages and deteriorates.

Minor aches and pains, caused by nervous tension, can be soothed and massaged away as the sense of relaxation sweeps over them.

Other clients merely like to be pampered, soothed and being made to feel beautiful. They enjoy having their bodies looked after and kept in trim.

Many like the pleasant sensory effect that massage can give. Feeling refreshed, invigorated, glowing and marvellous, for whatever reason, at the end of a treatment is the keynote that it has been successful.

Psychologically clients benefit, because they simply feel it is doing good, and this is why over the years the methods of massage have continually been improved.

Today, Peter Ling's teachings are still used, such as the passive movement. This is performed in the joint of a client, entirely by the therapist. It is neither assisted or resisted by any muscular activity of the client. These movements should always be given following a massage treatment, as they ensure mobility and progress.

Apart from the general body and beauty care massage, there are indications of massage in over a thousand conditions, affections and deformities. These must be diagnosed by a specialist and must not be treated, unless specific instructions are given.

THE CONTRA-INDICATIONS OF MASSAGE

This means the conditions in which it could be dangerous, or unwise to employ massage.

1. Increase of body temperature over 98.6°F or 37°C.

2. Any condition where pus is present, or around septic conditions.

3. Abnormal conditions of the skin i.e. burns, sores, syphilis, eczema, boils, carbuncles and skin diseases generally.

4. Circulatory diseases such as arterio-sclerosis, phlebitis, thrombosis and varicose veins.

5. Any unrecognizable lumps or swellings, cancers, tumours and tuberculosis.

6. Stones in the gall-bladder, kidney, ureter and bladder.

7. Any condition where there is an obvious danger of haemorrhage, like haemophilia, during a period or after the third month of pregnancy.
8. After recent bleeding from brain, bladder, lungs or stomach.
9. Acutely painful areas, over neuritis and neuralgia.
10. When glandular obesity is present.
11. Over unhealed and recently healed wounds and scars.
12. Loss of skin sensation.
13. Low blood pressure.
14. Grossly swollen limbs.
15. Acute inflammatory conditions, and rheumatoid arthritic conditions.
16. Abdominal massage should not be given in cases of diarrhoea, hernia or high blood pressure.
17. If a pacemaker is fitted, do not massage the abdomen, neck and shoulders.
18. If diabetes, avoid abdominal massage.

If in doubt about giving a massage, the client should always be referred to their GP.

In recent years, new techniques have come to the fore.

REMEDIAL MASSAGE
This is a deep tissue massage, used to stimulate circulation, release muscle spasm, and soften previously injured, restrictive tissues. Primarily for muscular problems and to treat specific conditions, i.e. sports injuries, disabled and immobile clients. Movements used are effleurage, frictions and vibrations.

SHIATSU
This originates from Japan. A form of massage using pressure application with fingers, thumbs, elbows, knees and sometimes, feet.

It is designed to work on the natural energy which flows along invisible lines, known as Meridians, or Energy Pathways.

When this natural energy flow becomes congested or blocked, symptoms of disease will result. The point of blockage is usually sensitive, or painful, to touch. It is similar, in principle, to Acupuncture.

NEURO-MUSCULAR

This massage was formulated in America and the Continent, primarily for use on muscles and nerves.

By working on the cutaneous sensory zones of the body, muscles can be loosened and relaxed. Particularly useful on the spinal channels where all the nerves emerge.

Petrissage movements are used to lift and release the large muscles of the back.

AROMATHERAPY MASSAGE ... WHAT IS IT?

Let's first recap on what we know about the effects of massage.

1. Circulation is accelerated. Arterial pressure is reduced and cardiac action is improved. It influences the distribution of blood, and increases the red and white cell content.
2. Promotes digestion, absorption and evacuation. Gastric and intestinal secretions are stimulated and hepatic function increased.
3. Increases body and local temperatures. Urine content is increased and the metabolic rate is accelerated.
4. Muscular system is nourished by better blood supply. Local heat removes fatigue products, burns up fat, restores tone and counteracts wastage.
5. Nervous system receives increased blood supply, which nourishes and removes fatigue products. Excites reflexes and exercises the whole system. Vitality of nerve trunks are renewed.
6. Nourishes and removes unwanted products from the skin.

Stimulates or numbs sensory nerve endings. Stimulates glandular function.

7. Influences the growth, maintenance, nourishment and normal repair to all tissues of the body.

With this in mind, aromatherapy massage treatments are for the harmony of mind, body and spirit, using pure, selected essential oils.

No particular massage routine is recognized as being the **ONE** to use for aromatherapy. Any massage which involves moving the hands over the skin, will help absorb the essential oil. So, any technique can be used as necessary, according to the client's needs.

The principles of aromatherapy are:

1. To transmit the Life-Force of the essential oils, so as to promote general health.

2. Working on circulation, lymphatics, muscles and nerves.

3. Working on energy pathways.

4. To use the best techniques available from the various types of massage.

Essential oils, often called the Essence of Life, help us in so many ways. They harmonize, purify, rejuvenate, restore and vitalize all cells and tissues of the body.

The essential oils' power of penetration through the skin is quite remarkable. Soluble in fatty parts of the skin, they quickly penetrate the different layers, to arrive in the bloodstream. Absorption time varies between twenty to seventy-five minutes.

The oils then work from within. Their effects are quick and powerful, so caution is required in their use.

By using the correct massage movements and selecting the appropriate essential oils all systems are improved.

1. Circulation is accelerated to capillary level. It aids the exchange of nutrition and gases between blood and cells.

2. Digestive secretions are increased, sluggish bowels stimulated and abdominal spasms are eased.

3. Muscular movements are improved and waste products eliminated. Fatigue and tiredness are reduced.
4. Nervous systems are harmonized and the equilibrium balanced.
5. Sweat glands, sebaceous glands and endocrine glands functions are regularized.
6. The skin's epidermis, dermis and connective tissue are stimulated and toned. Its natural colour, radiance and youth may also be restored.

THE HISTORY OF AROMATHERAPY

❦

Nowadays – Aromatherapy is as much a science as an art. The history of its science spans little more than a hundred years, but the history of its art began at least five thousand years ago.

Let's look back through some of the ancient records.

4500BC CHINA

The properties and benefits of aromatic herbs for the health of man were discovered in a medicinal book, as part of recommended treatments.

3000-1500BC EGYPT

Herbal essences were in common use. Egyptians offered aromatic oils to their Gods. Priests acted as spiritual healers, and also doctors. They used aromatic preparations as medicines and for embalming the dead. Incense and oils were used in religious ceremonies. Frankincense and Myrrh were highly rated and used for anointments of head and feet.

500BC INDIA

Fragrant Sandalwood was used in the building of Hindu temples. India produced an abundance of essential oils and had a barter agreement with Arabia.

370-285BC GREECE

Theophrastus, recorder of some interesting early thoughts on aromatic oils, mentioned that Greek perfumers worked in upper rooms, which did not face the sun, and were shaded as much as possible. For the sun, or a hot place, deprives the oils of their aromas and makes them lose their character. To this day we must be guided by this.

The Grecians used the oils as perfumes and care of the body. They were also given as medicines.

In the plague of Athens, the aromatics were used to fumigate the streets, to prevent the disease from spreading.

Hippocrates, known as the 'Father of Medicine' catalogued and described the benefits of at least three hundred plants.

50BC-200AD ROME

The Romans acquired their knowledge from the Greeks and, due to their conquests in various parts of the world, they were able to acquire a wide variety of essences.

Julius Caesar was known to favour baths perfumed with the oils, followed by a fragrant massage.

When Nero became Emperor of Rome perfumes and cosmetics were highly esteemed by his Court, as a result of their use by his wife. At her funeral Nero is said to have used more incense than Arabia could produce in ten years.

In his golden palace, the dining rooms were lined with movable ivory plates, concealing silver pipes which sprayed on the guests a stream of pleasant aromas.

At the fall of the Roman Empire, oils and perfumes lost their popularity.

900AD DARK AGES

During this time the Arabs also learnt about aromatherapy and several books were written. Avicenna, 'Prince of Physicians', succeeded in isolating from the rose some of its perfume in the form of an oil or otto, and was one of the first to produce rose water.

The Arabs have been credited with the invention of 'DISTILLATION' and became famous for their aromatic waters and essences.

1150AD
The advent of Lavender water. This is attributed to Saint Hildegard, a German Benedictine nun, although no formula was recorded.

1200AD
The Arabs passed their knowledge on to the Crusaders, particularly the distillation process. After the wars they brought back this knowledge to their own countries.

The Moors invaded Spain. Knowledge was passed on again, and this, in turn, passed into France.

The first importation of perfumes and essences by Britain were toilet preparations used by ladies of the harem, brought back by the Crusaders.

1450AD
The first European Medical Schools started. Herbalism and Aroma-therapy were studied.

All monasteries had their herbary and herbal books for reference. The old and the sick in their care were given herbal treatments.

1500AD
The Italians developed the art of extracting oils and the preparation of medicinal remedies. John Maria Farina, born 1685, an Italian, who emigrated to Cologne, created the first Eau de Cologne, a blend of citrus oils with lavender or rosemary, and is renowned for its refreshing qualities.

The perfume popularity spread through Europe to England. Queen Elizabeth I had her capes and footwear treated with oils and had oils sprinkled lavishly around the rooms.

Oils and aromatic preparations were sold for many reasons and uses, but chiefly to cover the smells from unwashed bodies.

1589AD

In Germany, a reference book listed approximately eighty oils with recommended uses. About this time Lavender essence was extracted for the first time.

1615AD

The earliest known formula for Lavender water is English. At this time there was tremendous interest in the treatments of disease by herbs, and it was proclaimed that every plant was associated by a spiritual bond to a particular disease.

1653AD

Nicholas Culpepper wrote his famous book, *The Complete Herbal*. Many still believe that the natural forces emanating from the astral bodies combined with the natural life-force within the plants, provide a basis for a very powerful form of healing.

1665AD

During the plague of London, in the reign of King Charles II, householders were advised to fumigate their rooms with aromatic essences in an attempt to fight the disease. Many people wore garlic, or cloves, or bunches of lavender around their necks for protection, and also to kill the smell of the dead. Surprisingly, the ones that did wear a herb seemed to survive the plague.

1808AD

Old account books record Napoleon as having ordered, for his personal use, sixty bottles of Eau de Cologne per month. He also ordered large quantities of aloes-wood. His favourite soap was

Brown Windsor, perfumed with a blend of Bergamot, Caraway, Cassia, Cedarwood, Clove, Lavender, Petitgrain, Rosemary and Thyme.

Empress Josephine preferred heavier odours, principally Musk.

1843AD

Towards the end of the Industrial Revolution, interest in herbal medicine began to wane. The science of chemistry was coming to the fore, with synthetic substances, both for medicine and cosmetic care.

1922AD

The Tomb of Tutankhamen at Luxor was opened by Howard Carter. A perfumed ointment of 1350 BC was found. This had a valerian-like fragrance, reminiscent of the Indian herb, NARD.

On analysis it was found to contain Frankincense. These two ingredients are known to be constituents of KYPHI, the most precious of all the perfumes of ancient Egypt.

1925AD

It was around this time the word aromatherapy was coined, to describe the usage of essential oils for healing purposes.

Modern aromatherapy begins with the work of Dr R.M. Gattefose, treating burns, gangrene and wounds during the First World War.

This continued until the advent of chloroform, drugs, medicine and surgery.

1937AD

After much research by the French chemist and scholar, a lengthy explanation of essential oil properties and methods of application was published in the book, *Aromatherapie*.

1964AD

Continuing in his footsteps, French Army Surgeon, Dr Jean Valnet, after further research, published, *The Practice of Aromatherapy*.

Another pioneer in the field, biochemist, Mme Marguerite Maury, translated these two works into modern times, extended her research and brought aromatherapy into the world of beauty, health and allied medicine.

EXTRACTION OF ESSENTIAL OILS

Essential oils are extracted from a particular part of the plant, for example:-

Bark/Resin - Benzion, Cinnamon, Frankincense, Myrrh

Berries/Seeds - Bay, Black Pepper, Caraway, Cardamom, Carrot, Coriander, Cypress, Fennel, Juniper, Parsley

Flowers - Basil, Camomile, Clary, Jasmine, Geranium, Lavender, Linden Blossom, Marigold, Marjoram, Melissa, Neroli, Rose, Ylang-Ylang

Fruits - Bergamot, Grapefruit, Lemon, Lime, Nutmeg, Orange, Tangerine

Leaves/Twigs - Bay, Cajuput, Clove, Eucalyptus, Geranium, Melissa, Patchouli, Peppermint, Petitgrain, Pine, Rosemary, Tea Tree, Violet

Roots/Grass - Citronella, Ginger, Lemongrass, Palmarosa, Vetivert

Whole Plant - Celery, Clary Sage, Sage, Thyme

Wood - Camphor, Cedarwood, Rosewood, Sandalwood

METHODS OF EXTRACTION

Enfleurage
This is chiefly applied to blossoms and petals that do not yield any appreciable amount of essential oil by steam or water distillation, or applied to flowers that are too delicate to be exposed to steam. Basically, a fatty surface is used to absorb the essential oil which is present in the flower petal. The petals are left for twenty-four hours, adhering to the fat, and then a new batch of petals is sprinkled on the same fat. Saturated fat, resulting from repeated treatments, is known as pomade. This is melted, and the essential oil is separated from the fat.

Distillation
Water and crushed plants are heated together until the oil vaporizes in the steam. The vapour is then cooled and a layer of essential oil floats on top of an aromatic water, i.e. Lavender water or Rose water.

Expression
The method used to extract oils that are found in the peel of ripe fruit. The most expensive, expressed oils are extracted by means of hand-rolling into sponges. For the cheaper method, whole fruit is crushed by machine, pure essential oil floats to the surface and carefully removed.

Maceration
This is a very old herbalist's method. The herb is immersed in a jar of vegetable oil, which is then put out in the sunlight. This is left for about two weeks, shaken daily, and then strained. Fresh herbs or plants are added and the process is repeated, until the required strength is achieved.

Solvent Extraction

The plant is crushed and covered with a solvent, such as acetone or ether. After the plants have been dissolved, the solvent is removed and a substance known as 'concrete' is left. A second solvent process then takes place. Pure ethanol removes most of the solvent and leaves an essential oil known as an absolute.

CHARACTERISTICS AND COMPOSITION OF ESSENTIAL OILS

۶ۍ

The essential oil within the growing plant has many purposes:
1. For reproduction – they attract insects to assist in this function.
2. For protection – they evaporate their essence against temperature extremes.
3. Chemical messages are used to warn other plants against invasion of insects and animals by means of scent and taste.
4. The oils help protect the plant against disease and help the plant repair itself.

All oils are:
   a) antiseptic, and most are anti-viral and anti-fungal
   b) heat and light sensitive
   c) volatile and flammable
   d) are soluble in carrier oils and alcohol, but only partially soluble in water
   e) are usually clear or pale coloured, and are liquid or semi-liquid, apart from German Camomile and Yarrow. Both are dark blue due to their Azulene content.

It is important to be aware of the exact location where plants bearing the healing oils are grown. All have different therapeutic properties. These can vary greatly area to area, and from year to year. Climate can influence the quality and their yield also varies. Storage in unsuitable conditions – too hot, too long – can ruin a good quality and render it useless.

ESSENTIAL OIL COMPOSITION

Plant oils are organic compounds and are variable in quality. Their structure is volatile and oxidise readily. The compounds are made up in different groups, each group having its own therapeutic properties.

1. *Aldehydes*

   These are antiseptic, pain relieving and anti-inflammatory.

2. *Coumarins*

   These compounds are found in all the citrus oils, except Mandarin. They are photo-toxic. Sun bathing and sun beds are not recommended after treatment, as blistering and pigmentation could occur.

3. *Esters*

   These are anti-fungal and anti-spasmodic. They soothe and calm the central nervous system.

4. *Ketones*

   Excellent for treating skin problems and respiratory conditions. They work on the mucous membranes.

5. *Oxides*

   Antiseptic and warming. Stimulates the digestive tract and helps the circulatory process.

6. *Phenols*

   Extra strong antiseptic. Care must be taken, as it is both an irritant and a stimulant. Could be toxic, if allowed to accumulate in the tissue.

7. *Terpene Alcohols*

   Found abundantly in the oils. Stimulating, uplifting, anti-viral and of low toxicity.

   A genuine plant oil can contain up to two hundred identifiable components, and many trace elements which are unidentified, and this makes it impossible to copy the formula. Synthetics have no place in aromatherapy treatments, as they have no therapeutic qualities whatsoever, and there is also a risk of allergies.

High altitude plants are purer and of far better quality than those grown in lower lying areas, as there is less contamination and pollution. The exact source of essential oils should be known before purchasing i.e. country of origin and whether organically grown. Modern growing methods tend to use fertilisers and pesticides. Unfortunately, these affect the essential compounds of the plant which, in turn, affect the pure essential oil.

The European herbs and plants grown in the pathway of the Chernobyl nuclear disaster have probably suffered in the aftermath. Not only has the essential oil suffered, but the soil will be contaminated for many years to come.

BOTTLE LABELLING AND OIL STORAGE

Everyone in the essential oil industry has a responsibility in the therapy's future, ensuring that bottles are labelled correctly and contain the following information:
1. Country of origin   e.g. Turkey
2. Purity   e.g. Pure 100% Essential Oil
3. Latin Name   e.g. Lavendula Angustifolia
4. Contents   e.g. 10ml/12ml/20ml
5. If not pure it should state – Diluted in carrier oil e.g. Sweet Almond
6. Very important – it should carry the use by date e.g. 6/2001
7. Warnings of their adverse effects
8. Not to be taken internally
9. Keep away from children
10. Do not use neat on the skin, unless otherwise directed
11. Dilute before use
12. Contains no additives
13. Sealed tamper-proof amber glass bottles
14. Price will indicate quality

Essential oils do not have an indefinite shelf life. Most oils will last approximately twenty-four months. The citrus oils will last approximately six months, if stored correctly, in ideal conditions, in amber glass bottles with tight fitting caps, preferably upright in a cool dark storage case or cupboard.

A discoloured, or cloudy, sour smelling oil has definitely gone off and should not be used. The shelf life of oils is reduced once blended to around three months maximum. This can be extended to six months if 10% wheatgerm oil is added to the blend.

BASE OR CARRIER OILS

When selecting the carrier oil, always check that it is a cold pressed vegetable oil for its purity and therapeutic values.

Carrier oils and their characteristics:

Apricot Kernel   - Very light texture, easily absorbed. Ideal for facial massage, excellent for mature skin.

Avocado   - Dark green in colour, extracted from the avocado pulp. Regenerative, contains Vitamins A and B. Excellent for stretch mark prevention.

Borage   - Very rich oil, good for mature skins. Restorative, anti-depressant, anti-inflammatory, diuretic and soothing.

Camellia   - Japanese oil, very good for the nervous tissues of skin and hair.

Evening Primrose - Very stimulating and regenerative. Contains Vitamins E and F. Good for ageing skin, eczema, psoriasis.

Grapeseed   - Very light fine oil. Contains vitamins and minerals. Highly penetrative. Ideal for oily skins.

Hazel Nut   - Light textured oil. Slightly astringent. Good for oily skins.

Jojoba   - Not really an oil, but a liquid wax. Excellent for troubled skins. Contains Vitamin E, protein and minerals.

Kiwi Seed   - Very light textured oil. Good for ageing skins, regenerative.

Olive	-	Suitable for all skin types. Medium texture, readily absorbed. Good for maturing skin, scar tissue, stretch marks.
Passion Flower	-	Fine textured oil. Ideal for irritated skin. Anti-inflammatory, anti-spasmodic, soothing, Vasco-protective and helps promote restful sleep.
Peach Kernel	-	Very rich textured oil. Contains Vitamin A. Prevents dehydration.
Rose Hip	-	Regenerative oil for burns, premature ageing and scars.
Sesame	-	Fine textured oil. Contains vitamins, minerals and Lecithin. Useful sun filter.
Soya Bean	-	Medium textured oil. Contains vitamins and minerals. Can cause allergic reaction.
Sunflower	-	Light textured oil, suitable for all skin types. Neutral oil, close to human sebum. Most economical.
Sweet Almond	-	Medium textured, suits all skin types. Very nourishing, rich in vitamins and minerals.
Walnut	-	High in unsaturated fatty acids. Wonderful for body massage.
Wheatgerm	-	Rather thick consistency. Excellent for ageing skins, stretch marks, scars etc. Check before use – could cause allergic reaction. 10% may be added to other carrier oils, as it is an anti-oxidant, it extends the shelf life of any blend.

Further useful oils:

Arnica	-	for sprains and bruising.
Calendula	-	anti-inflammatory for burns, wounds, ulcers.
Carrot	-	rich in flavonoids, ideal for skin problems.
Comfrey	-	reduces swelling, promotes healing in fractures.

Echinacea	–	powerful stimulant, anti-viral properties. Good for respiratory infections.
Kukui	–	deeply penetrative and healing.
St John's Wort	–	anti-bacterial, anti-viral, bruises, ulcers, varicose veins. Used to treat child bed-wetting and nightmares.

Some of these carrier oils have their own distinctive aromas. Always check that you agree with the smell, and that the essential oils *chosen* will blend harmoniously.

ESSENTIAL OILS A-Z

❧

There are over four hundred essential oils produced commercially and, as yet, many of them are not known for their therapeutic properties.

Following are a number of essential oils which have been chosen for their popularity and their healing benefits.

BASIL

LATIN NAME: OCIMUM BASILICUM
PLANT PART: WHITE FLOWERING TOPS
EXTRACTION: DISTILLATION
SOURCE: BULGARIA, COMORO ISLES, FRANCE
OIL COLOUR: PALE YELLOW/GREEN
AROMA: SWEET SPICY
SAFETY FACTORS: Do not use during pregnancy. Not for use on
                       children under 12. Could irritate sensitive skin.
                       Also known as Sweet Basil

THERAPEUTIC USE: CATARRH
                       CHEST INFECTIONS
                       CLEARS THE MIND
                       COLDS
                       COMBATS FEVER
                       COUGHS
                       DIGESTIVE PROBLEMS
                       INFLUENZA
                       INSECT REPELLENT
                       INSOMNIA
                       LOSS OF SMELL
                       MIGRAINE
                       MIND STIMULANT
                       MUSCLE SPASMS
                       NERVE TONIC
                       NERVOUS FATIGUE
                       POOR CONCENTRATION
                       SINUS CONGESTION
                       UPLIFTING
                       WEAK MEMORY

The action of Basil is usually enhanced when blending it with oils such as Bergamot, Lavender, Lemon, Mandarin or Orange.

N.B. Put 2-3 drops on a tissue and inhale. It is excellent if taking an examination, going on a long car journey, or having to concentrate for long periods. The mind is stimulated and the mental powers are revitalized.

BENZOIN

LATIN NAME:	STYRAX BENZOIN
PLANT PART:	RESIN, from deep cut in tree trunk
EXTRACTION:	SOLVENT
SOURCE:	JAVA, MALAYSIA, SUMATRA
OIL COLOUR:	DARK GOLDEN BROWN
AROMA:	SWEET VANILLA-LIKE
SAFETY FACTORS:	Not for Asthmatics. May irritate sensitive skins. Also known as Friars Balsam.

THERAPEUTIC USE:

ARTHRITIS
BED SORES
CATARRH
CHEST INFECTIONS
DIURETIC
ECZEMA
FROST BITE
GOUT
HIGHLY RELAXING
INFLAMMATORY CONDITIONS
IRRITATED SKINS
POOR CIRCULATION
PSORIASIS
RHEUMATISM
UPLIFTING

BLENDS WELL WITH: Eucalyptus, Lavender, Rose or Sandalwood

BERGAMOT

LATIN NAME:	CITRUS BERGAMIA
PLANT PART:	PEEL
EXTRACTION:	COLD EXPRESSION OF RIPE FRUIT
SOURCE:	ITALY, SICILY
OIL COLOUR:	DARK GREENISH BROWN
AROMA:	SWEET, SPICY, LEMONY
SAFETY FACTORS:	Photo-toxic. Do not use in the sun, or with UVA. Can irritate sensitive skins. Also known as 'The Happy Oil'. Excellent for vaporizing.

THERAPEUTIC USES:

ACNE
AIDS PRODUCTION OF URINE
ANTISEPTIC
ANTIVIRAL
COLD SORES
ECZEMA
FLATULENCE
GASTRIC STIMULANT
HEALS WOUNDS
OILY SKIN
POWERFULLY UPLIFTING
PSORIASIS
RESPIRATORY TRACT INFECTIONS
SOOTHING
URINARY TRACT INFECTIONS
VARICOSE ULCERS

BLENDS WELL WITH: Clary Sage, Cypress, Jasmine, Juniperberry, Lavender, Rosewood or Sandalwood

N.B. Invaluable for Anxiety, Tension and Worry.

BLACK PEPPER

LATIN NAME:	PIPER NIGRUM
PLANT PART:	CRUSHED BLACK PEPPERCORNS
EXTRACTION:	DISTILLATION
SOURCE:	INDIA
OIL COLOUR:	GREENISH YELLOW
AROMA:	WARMING, WOODY, SPICY, PEPPERY
SAFETY FACTORS:	Safe

THERAPEUTIC USES:

AIDS MUSCLE TONE
CATARRH
COLDS
DIGESTIVE STIMULANT
HAYFEVER
MUSCULAR ACHES/PAINS
POOR CIRCULATION
SORE THROAT
TONIC FOR THE SPLEEN

BLENDS WELL WITH:

Frankincense, Lavender, Rosemary or Sandalwood

CAMOMILE

෨෪

LATIN NAME:	MATRICARIA RECUTICA (GERMAN)
	ORMENIS MULTICAULIS (MOROCCAN)
	ANTHEMIS NOBILIS (ROMAN)
PLANT PART:	FLOWER HEADS
EXTRACTION:	DISTILLATION
SOURCE:	EUROPE, NORTH AFRICA, SOUTHERN GERMANY, USA
OIL COLOUR:	DARK INKY BLUE (GERMAN)
	PALE LEMON/GREEN (MOROCCAN/ROMAN)
AROMA:	SWEET, SMOOTH, HERBY
SAFETY FACTORS:	Very strong, but safe. The three varieties medicinal properties tend to overlap, but always use Roman Camomile for babies and children.

THERAPEUTIC USES:

ABSCESSES
ACNE
ALLERGIES
ANTI-SPASM
ANXIETY
ARTHRITIS (at every stage)
COLIC
COUGHS
CYSTITIS
DECONGESTANT
DEPRESSION
DERMATITIS
DIARRHOEA
DIGESTIVE UPSETS
ECZEMA
FACIAL NEURALGIA
GOUT
HAIR RINSE (for fair hair)
HAYFEVER
HEADACHE

HIGHLY SOOTHING
HOT FLUSHES
INFLAMMATORY CONDITIONS
INFLUENZA
INSOMNIA
IRRITABLE BOWEL
LOW BACK PAIN
MIGRAINE
NAUSEA
PAIN RELIEVING
PMT
RHEUMATIC CONDITIONS
SENSITIVE SKIN
SINUSITIS
SKIN ULCERS
STRESS RELATED CONDITIONS
TOOTHACHE
VERTIGO

BLENDS WELL WITH: Geranium, Lavender, Patchouli, Rose or
Ylang-Ylang

N.B. Very good for the highly strung, living on their nerves, and straining
their energies to the limit.

CEDARWOOD

❧

LATIN NAME:	CEDRUS ATLANTICA
PLANT PART:	WOOD CHIPS
EXTRACTION:	DISTILLATION
SOURCE:	NORTH AMERICA
OIL COLOUR:	YELLOW/ORANGE
AROMA:	SWEET BALSAMIC UNDERTONES
SAFETY FACTORS:	Not to be used during pregnancy. Can irritate sensitive skin

THERAPEUTIC USES:
ACNE
ALOPECIA
ASTHMA
BRONCHITIS
CATARRH
CIRCULATORY STIMULANT
COUGHS
DANDRUFF
ECZEMA
FALLING HAIR
RELATED KIDNEY/BLADDER PROBLEMS
RELAXING
RESPIRATORY TRACT INFECTIONS
RHEUMATIC PAINS
SKIN ERUPTIONS

BLENDS WELL WITH: Bergamot, Clary Sage, Eucalyptus, Jasmine, Juniperberry, Lavender or Rosemary

N.B. Excellent for vaporizing, to calm anxiety and nervous tension, also aids meditation.

CINNAMON LEAF

৵৻

LATIN NAME:	CINNAMONIUM ZEYLANICUM
PLANT PART:	LEAVES
EXTRACTION:	DISTILLATION
SOURCE:	INDIA, SKI LANKA
OIL COLOUR:	DEEP YELLOW/ORANGE
AROMA:	WARM, SPICY, HAUNTING
SAFETY FACTORS:	Use with care on sensitive skins. Must be well diluted in combination with other oils

THERAPEUTIC USES:
ANTI-BACTERIAL
ANTI-VIRAL
BRONCHITIS
CARMINATIVE
COLDS
COUGHS
DEPRESSION
INFLUENZA
MILD APHRODISIAC
RELAXING
STRESS RELATED CONDITIONS

BLENDS WELL WITH:
Camomile, Geranium, Ginger, Lavender, Mandarin, Patchouli or Sandalwood

CLARY SAGE

❧

LATIN NAME:	SALVIA SCLAREA
PLANT PART:	FLOWERING TOPS
EXTRACTION:	DISTILLATION
SOURCE:	FRANCE, USA
OIL COLOUR:	CLEAR PALE YELLOW
AROMA:	SWEET HERBACEOUS
SAFETY FACTORS:	Not to be used during pregnancy. Must not be used with Alcohol. Can cause drowsiness, best not to drive after use.

THERAPEUTIC USES:

ACHES/PAINS
ALL ROUND PANACEA
APHRODISIAC
ENCOURAGES HAIR GROWTH
EUPHORIC
EXHAUSTION
FRIGIDITY
HEADACHES
INSOMNIA
IRRITABILITY
LOWERS BLOOD PRESSURE
MUSCLE CRAMP
PMT
REGULATES HORMONES
RELAXING
RELIEVES STRESS
RESTORATIVE
SORE THROAT
UTERINE TONIC
VERTIGO

BLENDS WELL WITH: All Citrus Oils, Cedarwood, Jasmine, Juniperberry, Lavender, Rose or Sandalwood

N.B. Helps when there is a difficulty in accepting changes in life, such as children, home or occupation.

CYPRESS

ᴥ

LATIN NAME:	CUPRESSUS SEMPERVIRENS
PLANT PART:	CONES, NEEDLES, TWIGS
EXTRACTION:	DISTILLATION
SOURCE:	FRANCE, SPAIN
OIL COLOUR:	PALE YELLOW/GREEN
AROMA:	SWEET, WOODY, BALSAMIC
SAFETY FACTORS:	Safe

THERAPEUTIC USES:
ANTI-SPASMODIC
ASTHMA
BRONCHITIS
CONTRACTS BLOOD VESSELS
COUGHS
EXCESSIVE MENSTRUAL FLOW
HAEMORRHOIDS
HEALS WOUNDS
LIVER TONIC
MENOPAUSAL SYMPTOMS
PMT
POOR CIRCULATION
VARICOSE VEINS

BLENDS WELL WITH: Frankincense, Juniperberry, Lavender, Lemon, Neroli or Pine

N.B. Put 2-3 drops on a tissue or vaporize. This helps to control the fear of what others think.

EUCALYPTUS

❧

LATIN NAME: EUCALYPTUS GLOBULUS
PLANT PART: LEAVES, TWIGS
EXTRACTION: DISTILLATION
SOURCE: AUSTRALIA, PORTUGAL, SPAIN
OIL COLOUR: CLEAR TO PALE YELLOW
AROMA: PENETRATING, CAMPHORACEOUS, WOODY
SAFETY FACTORS: Do not use with Homeopathic Remedies

THERAPEUTIC USES: ALL RESPIRATORY CONDITIONS
                    ARTHRITIS
                    BALANCES BLOOD SUGAR
                    COLD SORES
                    CYSTITIS
                    DIARRHOEA
                    GOUT
                    INFLAMMATORY CONDITIONS
                    INFLUENZA
                    INSECT REPELLENT
                    MUSCULAR ACHES/PAINS
                    NEURALGIA
                    PAIN RELIEVING
                    POWERFUL ANTISEPTIC
                    VIRAL INFECTIONS

BLENDS WELL WITH: Benzoin, Cedarwood, Lavender, Marjoram, Pine
                    or Rosemary

N.B. Aids concentration. Balances extreme moods. Strong anti-viral,
      invaluable for most respiratory infections

FENNEL

&

LATIN NAME:	FOENICULUM VULGARE VAR DULCE
PLANT PART:	CRUSHED SEEDS
EXTRACTION:	DISTILLATION
SOURCE:	FRANCE
OIL COLOUR:	CLEAR
AROMA:	SWEET, ANISEED-LIKE
SAFETY FACTORS:	Safe. Can be used as a carminative, especially for children.

THERAPEUTIC USES:
ANTISPASMODIC
CONSTIPATION
DIGESTION
EXPECTORANT
MENOPAUSAL PROBLEMS
NATURAL COUGH MIXTURE
OBESITY

BLENDS WELL WITH: Black Pepper, Geranium, Lavender, Rose or Sandalwood

N.B. Helps to relieve flatulence and constipation, if used in abdominal massage.

FRANKINCENSE

೩ಒ

LATIN NAME:	BOSWELLIA CARTERI
PLANT PART:	RESIN
EXTRACTION:	DISTILLATION
SOURCE:	AFRICA
OIL COLOUR:	CLEAR
AROMA:	BEAUTIFUL RICH, BALSAMIC
SAFETY FACTORS:	Safe. Also known as Olibanum

THERAPEUTIC USES:
ACNE SCARRING
AGEING SKIN
BLEMISHED SKIN
DERMATITIS
EXCELLENT FOR ALL MUCOUS CONDITIONS
EXCELLENT SKIN CARE QUALITIES
HAEMORRHOIDS
HEALING
INDIGESTION
INFLAMMATORY CONDITIONS
LUNG TONIC
NERVOUS TENSION
RESPIRATORY CONGESTION
WRINKLES

BLENDS WELL WITH: Basil, Black Pepper, Juniperberry, Orange, Petitgrain or Sandalwood

N.B. Vaporize to aid meditation and spiritual development. It also helps to comfort those who find physical contact difficult and helps relieve mental fatigue.

GERANIUM

❧

LATIN NAME: PELARGONIUM GRAVEOLENS
PLANT PART: FLOWERS, LEAVES, STEMS
EXTRACTION: DISTILLATION
SOURCE: ALGERIA, CHINA, EGYPT, SPAIN
OIL COLOUR: YELLOW/GREEN
AROMA: DEEP SWEET, ROSY, FLORAL
SAFETY FACTORS: Safe. Also known as Rose Geranium

THERAPEUTIC USES: ALL SKIN TYPES
                     ANTI-COAGULANT
                     ATHLETES FOOT
                     BALANCES EXTREME MOODS
                     BROKEN CAPILLARIES
                     BRUISES
                     BURNS
                     CIRCULATION
                     CONGESTED, OILY SKIN
                     DRY ECZEMA
                     FATIGUE
                     FLUID RETENTION
                     FROST BITE
                     FUNGAL INFECTIONS
                     HORMONAL REGULATOR – due to oil stimulating
                     the adrenal cortex
                     INFLAMMATORY CONDITIONS
                     INSECT REPELLENT
                     LIVER/KIDNEY TONIC
                     LYMPHATIC CONGESTION
                     MENOPAUSE, balances oestrogen levels
                     NERVOUS TENSION
                     NEURALGIA
                     PMT
                     REGULATES HORMONE SYSTEM (during puberty)
                     SINUSITIS

SKIN DISORDERS
ULCERATED WOUNDS
UPLIFTING

BLENDS WELL WITH: Basil, Bergamot, Lavender, Rose, Rosemary or
                      Rosewood

N.B. 2-3 drops on a tissue and inhale. It calms acute fright when rigid with
     fear, or when an emergency arises. It has an harmonising effect,
     excellent for emotional extremes.

GINGER

ॐ

LATIN NAME:	ZINGIBER OFFICINALIS
PLANT PART:	DRIED ROOTS
EXTRACTION:	DISTILLATION
SOURCE:	CHINA, WEST INDIES
OIL COLOUR:	PALE YELLOW/GREEN
AROMA:	WARM, WOODY, SPICY, GINGERY
SAFETY FACTORS:	Slightly Photo-toxic

THERAPEUTIC USES:

ARTHRITIS
BACKACHE
CARMINATIVE, prevents griping
CATARRH
COLDS
COUGHS
DIGESTIVE PROBLEMS
FATIGUE
FLATULENCE
INVIGORATING
MUSCULAR ACHES/PAINS
NAUSEA
PROMOTES BOWEL EVACUATION
PROMOTES PERSPIRATION
RESPIRATORY CONGESTION
SINUSITIS
SORE THROATS
STIMULATES CIRCULATION
TRAVEL SICKNESS
WARMING STIMULANT

BLENDS WELL WITH: Lavender, Lemon, Mandarin, Orange and
Rosewood

GRAPEFRUIT

LATIN NAME: CITRUS PARADISI
PLANT PART: PEEL OF FRESH FRUIT
EXTRACTION: COLD EXPRESSION
SOURCE: BRAZIL, USA, WEST INDIES
OIL COLOUR: PALE YELLOW/GREEN
AROMA: FRESH, SHARP CITRUS
SAFETY FACTORS: Slightly Photo-toxic

THERAPEUTIC USES: CAUSES CONTRACTION OF THE TISSUES
                     CELLULITE
                     COUNTERACTS POISONING
                     DEPRESSION
                     DIGESTIVE STIMULANT
                     DIURETIC
                     EXHAUSTION
                     GENERAL TONIC
                     INHIBITS GROWTH OF BACTERIA
                     MIGRAINE
                     MUSCLE FATIGUE
                     STIMULATES LYMPHATIC SYSTEM
                     UPLIFTING
                     WATER RETENTION

BLENDS WELL WITH: Camomile, Geranium, Lavender, Rose or
                     Sandalwood

JASMINE

LATIN NAME: JASMINUM OFFICINALE

PLANT PART: FRESH WHITE FLOWERS, picked by hand at dawn

EXTRACTION: SOLVENT

SOURCE: CHINA, EGYPT, INDIA

OIL COLOUR: DARK ORANGE BROWN

SAFETY FACTORS: Could cause allergic reaction on sensitive skins, due to solvent residue. Also known as 'The King of Flowers'

THERAPEUTIC USES: ANTI-DEPRESSANT
ANTI-SPASMODIC
APHRODISIAC
CONFIDENCE BOOSTER
ENLARGEMENT OF THE PROSTATE
INFLAMMATORY CONDITIONS
IRRITATED SENSITIVE SKINS
MENSTRUAL PROBLEMS
PREVENTS SCARRING
RESTORES SKIN ELASTICITY
STRENGTHENS CONTRACTIONS IN CHILDBIRTH
STRESS RELIEVER
UPLIFTING

BLENDS WELL WITH: All citrus oils, Lavender, Neroli, Rose, Rosewood and Sandalwood

JUNIPERBERRY

LATIN NAME:	JUNIPERUS COMMUNIS
PLANT PART:	FRESH BLACK RIPE BERRIES
EXTRACTION:	DISTILLATION
SOURCE:	CANADA, FRANCE, SWEDEN
OIL COLOUR:	CLEAR/FAINT LEMON
AROMA:	FRESH, SWEET
SAFETY FACTORS:	Do not use during pregnancy, or in cases of kidney malfunction. Use on the elderly with caution

THERAPEUTIC USES:
ACNE/OILY SKINS
ARTHRITIS
BLOOD PURIFIER
CARMINATIVE
COLIC
CRAMP
CYSTITIS
ECZEMA
FLATULENCE
HANGOVER
HAYFEVER
INCREASES EXCRETION OF URIC ACID
RHEUMATISM
SPORTS INJURIES
STIMULATES CIRCULATION
WATER RETENTION

BLENDS WELL WITH: Benzoin, Bergamot, Cedarwood, Frankincense, Rosemary, Rosewood or Sandalwood

N.B. It is a strengthener and supporter. Excellent for people in the caring professions.

LAVENDER (Various)

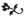

LATIN NAME:	LAVANDULA ANGUSTIFOLIA (ALPINE)
PLANT PART:	VIOLET BLUE FLOWERS, harvested early morning
EXTRACTION:	DISTILLATION, while still fresh
SOURCE:	FRENCH ALPS, PROVENCE
OIL COLOUR:	VERY PALE LEMON
AROMA:	VERY DEEP, SWEET FLORAL
SAFETY FACTORS:	Safe, high ester, low camphor content
LATIN NAME:	LAVANDULA ANGUSTIFOLIA (FRENCH) SAME SPECIES AS ALPINE, BUT GROWN AT A LOWER ALTITUDE Safe, low ester, high camphor content
LATIN NAME:	LAVANDULA OFFICINALIS (ENGLISH)
SOURCE:	NORFOLK, UK
OIL COLOUR:	PALE YELLOW
AROMA:	FLORAL, SLIGHTLY CAMPHORY
SAFETY FACTORS:	Safe
FURTHER SPECIES:	LAVANDULA VERA (DUTCH) It is thought to be a form of spike – not of therapeutic use
	LAVANDULA LATIFOLIA/SPICA (SPIKE LAVENDER) Produces spike or aspic oil. Contains fewer esters. Used chiefly as an insecticide and in industry
	LAVANDULA INTERMEDINFRAGRANS (LAVANDIN) A hybrid created by insects, highly scented. SOURCE: FRANCE, ITALY, SPAIN OIL COLOUR: YELLOW TO DARK YELLOW AROMA: CAMPHORY, HERBLIKE Used in soaps, talcums and household goods. Often sold as Lavender, but at a third of the price

THERAPEUTIC USES:
ACNE
ANTI-DEPRESSANT
ANTI-RHEUMATIC
BALANCES MIND AND BODY
BRUISES
BURNS
CHILBLAINS
COLDS, can be used during pregnancy
CYSTITIS
DIGESTIVE PROBLEMS
DIURETIC
FLUID RETENTION
FROST BITE
GOUT
HAIR LOSS
HEADACHES
HEAD LICE
HIGH BLOOD PRESSURE
IMMUNE SYSTEM STIMULATOR
INFLAMMATORY CONDITIONS
INFLUENZA
INSECT BITES
INSOMNIA
MIGRAINE
NERVOUS SYSTEM REGULATOR
PAIN RELIEVING
REJUVENATING AGENT
RELAXING
SCIATICA
SORE DRY THROAT
TRAVEL SICKNESS
VARICOSE VEINS
VERTIGO
WOUND HEALER

BLENDS WELL WITH:
Most oils, and especially with Bergamot,
Camomile and Geranium

N.B. Can be used for apprehensiveness, all forms of anxiety and tension,
panic and fear

LEMON

LATIN NAME:	CITRUS LIMON
PLANT PART:	FRESH PEEL
EXTRACTION:	COLD EXPRESSION
SOURCE:	FRANCE, ITALY, SPAIN, USA
OIL COLOUR:	PALE YELLOW/GREEN
AROMA:	FRESH, TANGY LEMON
SAFETY FACTORS:	Phototoxic, causes Dermatitis when exposed to UVA

THERAPEUTIC USES:
ACIDITY BALANCER
ACNE
ANAEMIA
ARRESTS BLEEDING
BROKEN CAPILLARIES
BRONCHITIS
CELLULITE
CLEARS SKIN OF DEAD CELLS
COLDS
CORNS
COUGHS
DETOXIFYING
DIGESTION STIMULANT
EXTERNAL BLEEDING
FLUID RETENTION
GARGLE
GREASY SKIN
INFLAMMATORY CONDITIONS
INSOMNIA
LARYNGITIS
LOWERS BLOOD PRESSURE
PMT
POOR CIRCULATION
STEMS NOSE BLEEDS
STIMULATES IMMUNE SYSTEM

BLENDS WELL WITH: Camomile, Geranium, Lavender, Neroli, Thyme
                      and Sandalwood

N.B. Very good for feelings of bitterness, jealousy and resentment.

LEMON GRASS

ೊಲ

LATIN NAME:	CYMBOPOGON FLEXUOSUS
PLANT PART:	GRASS
EXTRACTION:	DISTILLATION
SOURCE:	TROPICAL ASIA
OIL COLOUR:	YELLOW/LIGHT BROWN
AROMA:	EXCEEDINGLY LEMONY
SAFETY FACTORS:	Care should be taken – it could irritate the skin

THERAPEUTIC USES:

ACNE
ATHLETES FOOT
BOOSTS IMMUNE SYSTEM
COLITIS
ENTERITIS
EXCESSIVE PERSPIRATION
FLATULENCE
IMPROVES ENERGY
MAKES MUSCLES AND SKIN SUPPLE
POOR CIRCULATION
POOR DIGESTION DUE TO STRESS
SLACK SKIN TISSUE
TIRED LEGS
VENOUS CONDITIONS

BLENDS WELL WITH:

Geranium, Jasmine, Lavender, Rosemary and Vetivert

MANDARIN

LATIN NAME:	CITRUS RETICULATA
PLANT PART:	PEEL OF RIPE FRUITS
EXTRACTION:	COLD EXPRESSION
SOURCE:	SICILY, USA
OIL COLOUR:	AMBER/ORANGE
AROMA:	DEEP, SWEET MANDARIN
SAFETY FACTORS:	Safe

THERAPEUTIC USES:

ANXIETY
CALMS CARDIOVASCULAR SYSTEM
CONGESTED, OILY SKINS
CONSTIPATION
DELICATE CONSTITUTIONS
DEPRESSION
DIARRHOEA
DIGESTIVE TONIC
EMOTIONAL EMPTINESS
ENCOURAGES CIRCULATION
FLATULENCE
FOR CHILDREN
FOR THE ELDERLY
GASTRIC COMPLAINTS
HYPNOTIC
INSOMNIA
NERVOUSNESS
REVITALISING
SKIN TONIC
STRESS
STIMULATES BILE, LIVER AND STOMACH
UPLIFTING

BLENDS WELL WITH: Camomile, Geranium, Lavender, and Patchouli

N.B. Very popular as a room fragrance. Used in many hospices for its soothing effect.

MARJORAM

LATIN NAME: ORIGANUM MAJORANA LINNAEUS
PLANT PART: FLOWERING HEADS
EXTRACTION: DISTILLATION
SOURCE: FRANCE, SPAIN
OIL COLOUR: PALE LEMON
AROMA: SWEET, SMOOTH, SPICY, HERBY
SAFETY FACTORS: Do not use during pregnancy or if depressed

THERAPEUTIC USES: ACHES/PAINS
ANTI-SPASMODIC
BRONCHITIS
BRUISE DISPERSER
CHEST INFECTIONS
CONSTIPATION
DECONGESTANT
FLATULENCE
HEADACHES
HIGH BLOOD PRESSURE
INSOMNIA
INTESTINAL SPASMS
MENTAL STRAIN
MIGRAINE
MUSCLE RELAXANT
RELAXING
SINUSITIS

BLENDS WELL WITH: Bergamot, Cypress, Lavender, and Rosemary

N.B. Very soothing and deeply relaxing. Helps those who find it hard to show their emotions.

MELISSA

LATIN NAME: MELISSA OFFICINALIS
PLANT PART: FLOWERING TOPS, LEAVES
EXTRACTION: DISTILLATION
SOURCE: EUROPE
OIL COLOUR: PALE YELLOW
AROMA: WARM, LEMONY
SAFETY FACTORS: Do not use on children. Also known as 'The Elixir of Life', or Lemon Balm

THERAPEUTIC USES: ALLERGIES
                      ANAEMIA
                      ASTHMA
                      COUGHS
                      DEPRESSION
                      DIGESTIVE SYSTEM TONIC
                      HEADACHES
                      HEART TONIC
                      HIGH BLOOD PRESSURE REGULATOR
                      INSOMNIA
                      NERVOUS ANXIETY
                      PALPITATIONS
                      PMT
                      SHOCK TREATMENT
                      SOOTHES MIND AND BODY

BLENDS WELL WITH: Lavender, Geranium, Neroli, or Ylang-Ylang

MYRRH
🌿

LATIN NAME:	COMMIPHORA MYRRHA
PLANT PART:	RESIN
EXTRACTION:	DISTILLATION
SOURCE:	AFRICA, INDIA
OIL COLOUR:	AMBER
AROMA:	DEEP, STRONG BALSAMIC
SAFETY FACTORS:	Do not use during pregnancy. Do not use for prolonged periods.

THERAPEUTIC USES:

ACNE
CATARRH
DERMATITIS
FLATULENCE
FUNGAL INFECTIONS
GUM PROBLEMS
HAEMORRHOIDS
MOUTH ULCERS
SCAR TISSUE
SKIN PROBLEMS
THROAT PROBLEMS
ULCERATIONS
WOUNDS

BLENDS WELL WITH: Camomile, Lavender, Lemon, Neroli, Patchouli, and Rose

NEROLI

LATIN NAME:	CITRUS AURANTIUM
PLANT PART:	ORANGE BLOSSOM
EXTRACTION:	DISTILLATION/SOLVENT
SOURCE:	MEDITERRANEAN
OIL COLOUR:	PALE LEMON/ORANGE
AROMA:	LIGHT FLORAL, WOODY
SAFETY FACTORS:	Safe. Can be used during pregnancy. Ultra relaxing.

THERAPEUTIC USES:

ALL SKIN TYPES
ANXIETY
APHRODISIAC
DEPRESSION
INSOMNIA
MUSCLE SPASMS
PALPITATIONS
PMT
POOR CIRCULATION
REJUVENATING
RELAXING
SCAR TISSUE
SHOCK REMEDY
SKIN ELASTICITY IMPROVER
STRETCH MARKS

BLENDS WELL WITH: Benzoin, Clary Sage, Cypress, Geranium, Lavender, Rose, Rosewood or Sandalwood

N.B. It calms and soothes the body, mind and spirit. Excellent for stress related problems.

ORANGE

૱

LATIN NAME:	CITRUS SINENSIS
PLANT PART:	FRESH PEEL
EXTRACTION:	COLD EXPRESSION
SOURCE:	SPAIN, USA, WEST INDIES
OIL COLOUR:	YELLOW/ORANGE
AROMA:	SWEET, FRUITY-ORANGEY
SAFETY FACTORS:	Phototoxic. Not to be used with UVA

THERAPEUTIC USES:
AFTER SUN WRINKLES
BRONCHITIS
COLDS
CONSTIPATION
DEPRESSION
DERMATITIS
DULL, OILY SKIN
DYSPEPSIA
ECZEMA
FATIGUE
FLUID RETENTION
GASTRIC SPASM
MENOPAUSAL PROBLEMS
NERVOUS TENSION
PALPITATIONS
REJUVENATES AGEING SKIN
RELAXING
STRESS

BLENDS WELL WITH: Cinnamon, Frankincense and Lavender

N.B. Energises when lethargic. Helps when working under pressure.

PATCHOULI

LATIN NAME:	POGOSTEMON CABLIN
PLANT PART:	LEAVES
EXTRACTION:	DISTILLATION
SOURCE:	INDIA, INDONESIA, SOUTH AMERICA
OIL COLOUR:	DARK ORANGE/BROWN
AROMA:	RICH EARTHY, HERBY
SAFETY FACTORS:	Safe

THERAPEUTIC USES:

ACNE
ANXIETY
APHRODISIAC
BURNS
CRACKED, WEEPING SKIN CONDITIONS
DEPRESSION
ECZEMA
GENERAL SKIN CARE
HAEMORRHOIDS
INFLAMMATORY CONDITIONS
NERVOUS TENSION
PROMOTES THE FORMATION OF SCAR
    TISSUE
REJUVENATING
RINGWORM
UPLIFTING
WRINKLES

BLENDS WELL WITH: Bergamot, Geranium, Lavender, Myrrh, Neroli,
Pine and Rose

N.B. Has an exceedingly strong anti-depressant action.

PEPPERMINT

❧

LATIN NAME:	MENTHA PIPERITA
PLANT PART:	FLOWERING TOPS
EXTRACTION:	DISTILLATION
SOURCE:	CHINA, USA
OIL COLOUR:	PALE LEMON
AROMA:	STRONG GRASSY MINT
SAFETY FACTORS:	Safe. Do not use with Homeopathic Remedies, as it acts as an antidote. Never use undiluted or as a bath essence. Do not use at night, or alone as a massage oil.

THERAPEUTIC USES:

ACHING FEET
ACNE
ACTS QUICKER THAN ASPIRIN
AIDS CLEAR THINKING
ASTHMA
BLOOD CLEANSER
BRUISES
COLDS
COLIC
COOLING
CRAMP IN THE INTESTINES
DERMATITIS
DIGESTIVE PROBLEMS
DIARRHOEA
FAINTING
FOOD POISONING
HEADACHES
INFLAMMATORY CONDITIONS
INFLUENZA
IRRITABLE BOWEL
IRRITATION
LARYNGITIS
MENTAL FATIGUE

MIGRAINE
MOSQUITO BITES
MUSCULAR PAIN
NAUSEA
NEURALGIA
PAIN RELIEVING
PLEASANT MOUTHWASH
REGULATOR OF THE NERVOUS SYSTEM
SHOCK REMEDY
STOMACH PAINS
SUNBURN
TRAVEL SICKNESS
VERTIGO

BEST USED ALONE, but does blend with Juniperberry, Lavender and Rosemary.

N.B. Very soothing and deeply relaxing. Helps those who find it hard to show their emotions.

PETITGRAIN

ॐ

LATIN NAME:	CITRUS AURANTIUM
PLANT PART:	LEAVES, TWIGS
EXTRACTION:	DISTILLATION
SOURCE:	BRAZIL, FRANCE, PARAGUAY
OIL COLOUR:	PALE LEMON/AMBER
AROMA:	FLOWERY CITRUS, EARTHY
SAFETY FACTORS:	Safe. Known as the 'Poor Man's Neroli'

THERAPEUTIC USES:

ACNE
ANXIETY
BACKACHE
DEPRESSION
GREASY SKIN/HAIR
INSOMNIA
NERVE SOOTHER
NERVOUS EXHAUSTION
STOMACH SOOTHER
STRESS
WATER RETENTION

BLENDS WELL WITH: Cedarwood, Ginger, Grapefruit, Patchouli, Rosewood and Sandalwood

PINE NEEDLE

❧

LATIN NAME: PINE SYLVESTRIS
PLANT PART: NEEDLES
EXTRACTION: DISTILLATION
SOURCE: SCANDINAVIA, USA
OIL COLOUR: CLEAR
AROMA: PINE BALSAMIC
SAFETY FACTORS: Safe

THERAPEUTIC USES: ACUTE/CHRONIC MUSCLE INJURIES
                   ARTHRITIS
                   CATARRH
                   EXHAUSTION
                   GOUT
                   INFLUENZA
                   INVIGORATING
                   MENTAL REVITALIZER
                   NEURALGIA
                   POOR CIRCULATION
                   RESPIRATORY CONDITIONS
                   RHEUMATISM
                   SINUSITIS
                   SORE THROATS
                   URINARY INFECTIONS

BLENDS WELL WITH: Cedarwood, Cypress, Eucalyptus, Lavender, and
                   Rosemary

ROSE

❧

LATIN NAME:	ROSE DAMASCENA
PLANT PART:	ROSE PETALS
EXTRACTION:	1. SOLVENT (ABSOLUTE)
	2. DISTILLATION (OTTO)
SOURCE:	BULGARIA, TURKEY
OIL COLOUR:	1. RICH RED/ORANGE
	2. ORANGE TO RED
AROMA:	1. ROUND HONEY ROSE
	2. SPICY ROSY, POWERFUL
SAFETY FACTORS:	Safe – least toxic of all oils. Known as 'The Queen of Oils'

THERAPEUTIC USES:

ALL SKIN TYPES
ANOREXIC PROBLEMS
ANTI-VIRAL
BROKEN CAPILLARIES
DEPRESSION
FRIGIDITY
HEART TONIC
HELPS REDUCE CHOLESTEROL IN BLOOD
    STREAM
INFLAMMATORY CONDITIONS
INSOMNIA
LIVER TONIC
LOSS OF APPETITE
MENOPAUSAL SYMPTOMS
PMT
RESPIRATORY PROBLEMS
SEX ORGANS TONIC
SKIN ULCERS
SOOTHING TO THE NERVOUS SYSTEM
STOMACH TONIC

BLENDS WELL WITH: Bergamot, Clary Sage, Geranium, Jasmine, Patchouli, Rosewood and Sandalwood

ROSEMARY

さん

LATIN NAME:	ROSMARINUS OFFICINALIS
PLANT PART:	FLOWERING TOPS
EXTRACTION:	DISTILLATION
SOURCE:	FRANCE, SPAIN, USA
OIL COLOUR:	CLEAR
AROMA:	PENETRATING, MINTY, HERBY
SAFETY FACTORS:	Not to be used on Epileptics. Do not use during pregnancy.
THERAPEUTIC USES:	ACHES/PAINS

ACHES/PAINS
ASTHMA
BLOOD AND LYMPH CLEANSER
BLOOD PRESSURE HIGH AND LOW REMEDY, due
   to the effects on the tension of the blood
   vessels
BOOSTS CIRCULATION, LIVER AND KIDNEY
   FUNCTION
CONSTIPATION
DANDRUFF INHIBITOR
DEPRESSION
HANGOVERS
HEADACHES
HEART TONIC
HELPS TO LOWER BLOOD CHOLESTEROL
LIVER AND GALL BLADDER TONIC
MENTAL FATIGUE
MUSCLE FATIGUE
NERVOUS SYSTEM TONIC
PAIN RELIEVING
RELIEVES SPASM OF THE DIGESTIVE TRACT
RESPIRATORY PROBLEMS
RHEUMATISM
STIMULATES FAILING MEMORY
SCALP TONIC FOR BALDING AND FALLING HAIR
WATER RETENTION

BLENDS WELL WITH: Basil, Citrus Oils, Juniperberry, Lavender,
                      Rosewood and Thyme.

N.B. Good for feelings of inadequacy and disorientation. Clears the head
and clarifies the thoughts.

ROSEWOOD

æ

LATIN NAME:	ANIBA ROSAEODORA VAR AMAZONICA
PLANT PART:	WOOD CHIPPINGS
EXTRACTION:	DISTILLATION
SOURCE:	BRAZIL, SOUTH AMERICA
OIL COLOUR:	CLEAR
AROMA:	SWEET, WOODY, SPICY, ROSE-LIKE
SAFETY FACTORS:	Safe. Also known as Bois de Rose

THERAPEUTIC USES:
ACNE
AGEING SKIN PIGMENTATION
ANTI-DEPRESSANT
BALANCING AND STABILIZING
BOOSTS THE IMMUNE SYSTEM
CELL AND TISSUE STIMULANT
DERMATITIS
ECZEMA
FRIGIDITY
HEADACHES
HELPFUL FOR CHRONIC COMPLAINTS
IMPOTENCE
INSECT REPELLENT
NERVOUS TENSION
REJUVENATING
SCAR TISSUE
SOOTHING
STRETCH MARKS
THROAT INFECTIONS
WRINKLES

BLENDS WELL WITH: Camomile, Geranium, Jasmine, Lavender, Neroli, Orange, Rose and Ylang-Ylang

N.B. Good for inner tension and when over-critical of others.

SANDALWOOD

LATIN NAME: SANTALUM ALBUM
PLANT PART: HEARTWOOD OF TRUNK
EXTRACTION: DISTILLATION
SOURCE: MYSORE REGION, EAST INDIA
OIL COLOUR: PALE YELLOW
AROMA: SMOOTH, SWEET, WOODY, HEAVY
SAFETY FACTORS: Safe. Also known as Bois de Santal

THERAPEUTIC USES: ABSCESSES
                       ACNE
                       AGEING SKIN
                       BOOSTS IMMUNE SYSTEM
                       BROKEN CAPILLARIES
                       CHEST COMPLAINTS
                       CRACKED DRY SKIN
                       CYSTITIS
                       DEPRESSION
                       DRY ECZEMA
                       HAS AN AFFINITY FOR THE URINARY TRACT
                       INSOMNIA
                       IRRITATION
                       LYMPHATIC CONGESTION
                       MATURE SKIN
                       NERVOUS TENSION
                       SENSITIVE SKIN
                       SEXUAL STIMULANT
                       SORE THROAT
                       STRONG ANTISEPTIC PROPERTIES
                       TONSILLITIS

BLENDS WELL WITH: Benzoin, Cypress, Frankincense, Jasmine,
                       Lavender, Lemon, Neroli, Rose and Ylang-Ylang

N.B. Balancing for people who like their own way. Helpful for sexual
     anxiety. Aid to meditation and intuitive development. Also helps to
     give strength to the emotionally weak.

TEA TREE

$\partial\mathcal{L}$

LATIN NAME:	MELALEUCA ALTERNIFOLIA
PLANT PART:	LEAVES
EXTRACTION:	DISTILLATION
SOURCE:	AUSTRALIA
OIL COLOUR:	CLEAR
AROMA:	FRESH CAMPHOR, SPICY, PENETRATING
SAFETY FACTORS:	Safe

THERAPEUTIC USES:
ABSCESSES
ACNE
ACTIVATES THE WHITE BLOOD CELLS TO FIGHT
    INFECTION
ANTI-BACTERIAL, FUNGAL, VIRAL PROPERTIES
ATHLETES FOOT
BLISTERS
BOILS
BUNIONS
BURNS
CHEST INFECTIONS
CHICKEN POX RASH
CHILBLAINS
COLDS
COLD SORES
COMBATS BAD BREATH
CORNS
DRY SCALP
EAR INFECTIONS
GENITAL ITCHING
GYNAECOLOGICAL CONDITIONS
HEAD LICE
INFECTED FACIAL SPOTS
INSECT BITES/STINGS
INSECT REPELLENT
IMPETIGO
IRRITATING/ITCHY CONDITIONS

MOUTH/NOSE INFECTIONS
PNEUMONIA
PRURITIS
PSORIASIS
RINGWORM
SHINGLES
SINUSITIS
STIMULATES IMMUNE SYSTEM
THROAT INFECTIONS
THRUSH
TOE NAIL FUNGAL INFECTIONS
VERRUCAE
WARTS

BLENDS WELL WITH: Eucalyptus, Lavender, Peppermint and Rosemary

N.B. First Aid in a bottle. Best used alone. Excellent for feelings of
uncleanliness. It refreshes and revitalises; use on tissue or vaporize.

THYME

𝕤𝕖

LATIN NAME:	THYMUS VULGARIS
PLANT PART:	RED FLOWERING TOPS
EXTRACTION:	DISTILLATION
SOURCE:	SPAIN, USA
OIL COLOUR:	YELLOW/ORANGE
AROMA:	WARM, PENETRATING, SPICY
SAFETY FACTORS:	Do not use during pregnancy. Do not use if kidney function is impaired

THERAPEUTIC USES:
ACHES/PAINS
ANAEMIA
ANTI-FUNGAL
ASTHMA
BACKACHE
BRUISES
FATIGUE
FEVER
FLATULENCE
INFLUENZA
NERVOUS EXHAUSTION
SCIATICA
SKIN INFECTIONS
SPRAINS
VERY EFFECTIVE ANTISEPTIC FOR USE IN
  VIRULENT DISEASES

BLENDS WELL WITH: Bergamot, Lavender, Lemon, Melissa and
Rosemary

N.B. Vaporized, it has an uplifting effect. Also helpful for exhaustion and
  nervous anxiety.

VETIVERT

LATIN NAME:	VETIVERIA ZIZANOIDES
PLANT PART:	CHOPPED ROOTS (GRASS)
EXTRACTION:	DISTILLATION
SOURCE:	CHINA, JAVA, SRI LANKA
OIL COLOUR:	AMBER/GREEN
AROMA:	DEEP EARTHY, RELAXING
SAFETY FACTORS:	Safe. Known as 'The Oil of Tranquillity'

THERAPEUTIC USES:

ACNE
ANXIETY
ARTHRITIS
CRAMP
DEEPLY RELAXING
EXTREMELY SOOTHING
INSOMNIA
MUSCLE INJURIES
NERVOUS TENSION

BLENDS WELL WITH: Camomile, Clary Sage, Geranium, Ginger, Jasmine, Lavender, Neroli, and Rosewood

N.B. Vaporized, it is extremely calming. Excellent for anxiety.

YLANG-YLANG EXTRA

❧

LATIN NAME:	CANANGA ODORATA VAR GENUINA
PLANT PART:	FLOWERS
EXTRACTION:	DISTILLATION
SOURCE:	COMORO ISLES
OIL COLOUR:	PALE YELLOW
AROMA:	DEEP, SWEET FLORAL, BALSAMIC
SAFETY FACTORS:	Safe, but can cause nausea in certain individuals. There are other distillations, but of lower therapeutic value.
THERAPEUTIC USES:	ACNE

ACNE
APHRODISIAC
CIRCULATORY SYSTEM TONIC
DANDRUFF
DEPRESSION
EUPHORIC
FRIGIDITY
GENERAL TONIC
HAIR PROBLEMS
HIGH BLOOD PRESSURE REGULATOR
HORMONE BALANCER
HYPOTENSIVE
IMPOTENCY
NERVOUS TENSION
PALPITATIONS
REGULATES ADRENALINE FLOW
REGULATES CARDIAC AND
    RESPIRATORY RHYTHM
RELAXANT
SENSUAL
SEXUAL PROBLEMS
SHOCK
STRESS
UPLIFTING

BLENDS WELL WITH: Clary Sage, Geranium, Jasmine, Lavender, Lemon, Rosewood and Sandalwood

N.B. Inhaled from a tissue, or vaporized, it helps calm anger and fear, frustration and irritability. It also helps heal the feeling of guilt, jealousy, resentment and selfishness.

HOW TO BLEND ESSENTIAL OILS

After reading through the list of essential oils, and their therapeutic use, you will find that several of these oils will treat the same condition.

Each one is correct. It is your choice of oil. Whichever aroma attracts you is the right one. Just follow your nose.

One essence may be added to the carrier oil, or a blend of two or three essences may be more suitable, to provide a good therapeutic effect.

If more essences are added to blend, it could well counteract the effect required.

When mixing a strong smelling oil with a weaker one, use three drops of the weaker, to one drop of the stronger.

The correct healthy adult strength should be 2½%

e.g.
50 ml bottle of carrier oil	=	25 drops
30 ml bottle of carrier oil	=	15 drops
25 ml bottle of carrier oil	=	12 drops
20 ml bottle of carrier oil	=	10 drops
15 ml bottle of carrier oil	=	7 drops
10 ml bottle of carrier oil	=	5 drops

The following measurements are a useful guide:-

20 drops essential oil	=	1 millilitre
200 drops essential oil	=	10 millilitres
5 millilitres	=	1 teaspoonful
10 millilitres	=	1 dessertspoonful
20 millilitres	=	1 tablespoonful

The best way to understand, and calculate your mix, is as follows: Take a 20 ml bottle of carrier oil and add 10 drops of your chosen essential oil.

Alternatively, take a 10 ml bottle of carrier oil and add 5 drops of your selected essential oil.

Or take a 5 ml teaspoonful of carrier oil and add 2 drops of essential oil.

These are the maximum number of drops which should be used.

If the number of drops do not work out to a round figure, use the lower number – e.g. 2½ drops – add 2 drops and not 3.

The essential oils work on the same principle as Homeopathy, where the tiniest quantity is effective.

Mixing more than one oil together is called blending. It is better to use a maximum of three; two oils to enhance and develop each others healing benefits, and the third to balance, or anchor, the blend.

Natural balancing oils are:

Geranium, Lavender, Neroli, Rose and Rosewood.

Any one of these will anchor any blend.

There is a very wide variety of methods in which the oils can be applied. Just as the properties and action of the essential oils vary, so does the way in which they can be used.

THE APPLICATION OF OILS

There are numerous ways to enjoy, and reap, the benefits from aromatherapy oils.

BATHS

Many conditions may be treated this way to help to reduce stress and encourage sleep. Five to six drops may be added to running water. Relax in the bath for at least 15-20 minutes for the oil to be absorbed, and to inhale the vapour. Full benefit will have been received from the medicinal and aromatic properties. Oils baths are a self-help for stress related illness.

COMPRESSES

Compresses can be used on areas that cannot, or must not, be massaged. When the condition is acute, apply a cold compress. For a chronic condition, apply a warm damp compress. Put 3-5 drops of essential oil into a bowl of cold, or hot, water. Take a ladies handkerchief and fold to the size required. Gently lay on the surface of the water. Allow the cotton to absorb the thin film of essential oil and squeeze out gently. For a limb, place the compress on the affected area, cover with cling film, then cover with a towel and leave 20-30 minutes.

DIRECT APPLICATION

In some circumstances, undiluted oils may be used:

BURNS	Use Lavender
COLD SORES and SHINGLES	Use Bergamot
VERRUCAE and WARTS	Use Tea Tree

Apply daily with cotton wool bud, taking care not to get the oil on the surrounding tissue.

HAND AND FOOT BATHS

Add 2-4 drops of oil to a bowl of water.

For a recent injury, cold water should be used with cooling oils, such as Camomile, Eucalyptus, Lemon and Peppermint.

For old injuries, use hot/warm water with warming oils, such as Benzoin, Black Pepper, Ginger, Rosemary and Thyme.

Arthritic hands and feet benefit by using the hot water method for chronic conditions and the cold water method for acute conditions. Allow to soak for 15-20 minutes.

N.B. Do not mix two cool oils or two warm oils together.

INHALATION

This method is beneficial for catarrh, colds, coughs, influenza, migraine, sinusitis and sore throats, using the oils of Benzoin, Basil, Eucalyptus, Lavender, Sandalwood or Tea Tree.

1. Place 2-3 drops of oil on a tissue and inhale as necessary.
2. Put 3-4 drops of oil in a bowl of steaming water, cover the head with a towel and inhale the steam for 5-10 minutes.

MASSAGE

Everyone can enjoy the luxury of a full body massage, or localized massage, with an aromatic blend of specially formulated oils. By concentrating on the main nerve points of the body, it allows physical absorption where it infuses cellular matter, acting as a stimulant to restore the body's rhythm. The effect of the fragrance, both mentally and physically, can induce a state of relaxation, relieving tension and making it easier to dispel traumas.

Massage and oils can make the powers of perception clearer and more acute, giving harmony to mind and body.

ROOM METHODS

These methods can create specific moods, or help to prevent the spread of air-borne diseases. They also help to boost the immune system, depending on the selection of oils chosen.

Various methods can be used as follows:

a) Oil burners are very popular. 1-2 drops put into water in a saucer can be placed over a night candle.

b) 1 drop of oil can be placed onto a cold light bulb. When the light is switched on, the fragrance is released.

c) 3-5 drops can be put onto a tissue, or cotton wool, and placed behind a radiator.

d) 3-4 drops of oil, added to a bowl of steaming water, vaporizes the oil and can be placed in any room.

e) Electric aroma stones are now available. Place 3-4 drops onto the stone, which is thermostatically heated, and enjoy the fragrance. Water may be added to extend vaporization times, and it can be left running unattended, or whilst you sleep.

f) Electric Aroma-Stream is a clean, effective and safe method of dispensing your oil's fragrance. No heat, naked flame or water is used, just a stream of air. Ideal for use with cough vapour remedies, and for use in the children's bedroom.

HOW WE SMELL AND ITS EFFECTS

The human mechanism for picking up, and differentiating between smells is a very delicate operation. Approximately twenty million olfactory receptor cells are situated in an area the size of a small coin in the roof of the nasal cavity, just beneath the eye sockets. Not only can these cells detect as many as 4,000 separate, and clearly identifiable aromas, but they only require a minute fraction of the essential oil to do so.

Aromas are created by moisture molecules evaporating into the atmosphere. All living matter and many inert things, give off their own separate invisible and highly volatile essences, whether it be the heady fragrance of Jasmine, or the acrid fumes from a car's exhaust system.

Most smells have very distinct properties – aromatic, fragrant, fruity, pungent, spicy or woody, but each individual will appreciate them differently.

Association, memory and perhaps anticipation, play an important part in determining whether we respond negatively or positively to certain smells.

Subconsciously these smells are catalogued away in the vast olfactory library of the brain, influencing mood to soothe, to invigorate, or even stupefy, if given in large enough doses.

In the summer of 1999, a team of scientists made a discovery while studying how pleasurable experiences affected the immune system. They found that the sense of smell is quite unique. It is directly wired into the left side of the brain, which controls the emotions.

Not only does it affect the body psychologically, but also physically. by changing the immune system.

Essential oils when blended, and perfumes are made up of Top, Middle and Base notes.

TOP NOTES
(These are all stimulating and uplifting)

This is the most volatile part of a fragrance. It has the most immediate effect on the sense of smell. It evaporates into the air in seconds; gives the first fleeting impression that lasts for about 15-20 minutes, but subsides as the lower notes start to develop.

MIDDLE NOTES
(These affect general metabolism and most body systems)

This is the heart of the fragrance. It melts and transforms the top note and carries the fragrance for about 30 minutes, whilst the base note starts to develop. This usually takes about 10-20 minutes and lasts up to 3-4 hours.

BASE NOTES
(These are the most soothing and relaxing)

These determine the holding power of a fragrance and it is the true characteristic for which the rest of the smell will be created. Initially strong and unpleasant smelling, base notes take approximately 30 minutes to develop their 'true' and beautiful smell. This aroma can linger for up to six hours once all evaporation has taken place. Sometimes a small residual part of it may remain for several weeks. This is known as the dry out.

Usually, essential oil treatments are used by normal healthy adults. However, they can also be used by the more vulnerable, like babies, children, pregnant women, the elderly and the terminally sick.

BABIES AND CHILDREN

UP TO THE AGE OF TWO MONTHS
The oils of Roman Camomile, Alpine Lavender and Mandarin are allowed. All babies love a gentle massage. Take 20 mls of Sweet Almond Oil and add 2 drops of a chosen essential oil. Apply with slow soothing effleurage movements and watch baby relax. Alternatively, put 1 drop of oil in the bath water, but only use once per week.

TWO MONTHS TO TWELVE MONTHS
Use the same dilution, but the range of essential oils may be extended to include Cypress, Eucalyptus and Tea Tree.

Roman Camomile is known as the 'children's oil'. Excellent for teething problems – apply a compress to the jaw. Also very good for nappy rash – apply a compress to the area using 1 drop of oil only. Tantrums and poor sleep patterns can also be helped by vaporizing 1 drop of oil in their nursery.

Cypress, Eucalyptus and Tea Tree are very good for coughs, sniffles and croup etc. Treat by vaporizing.

TWELVE MONTHS TO SEVEN YEARS
Increase the strength to 20 mls of carrier oil and add 4 drops of a selected essential oil.

SEVEN YEARS TO TWELVE YEARS
Increase the strength to 20 mls of carrier oil and add 6 drops of an essential oil.

OVER TWELVE YEARS

Increase to adult strength i.e. 20 mls of carrier oil and add 10 drops of a chosen essential oil.

DISABLED CHILDREN

Care must be taken when treating these children. Do not exceed 4 drops of essential oil, as the eliminatory system may be faulty, and the risk of oil toxicity may occur.

N.B. As essential oils are only partially soluble in water, it is advisable to dilute them in a carrier oil before bathing a baby or small child. Their skin is very delicate and if it came into contact with a minute molecule of essential oil, it could irritate quite badly. Also children have a tendency of splashing in the water, or even sucking their thumbs, and it could possibly get into their eyes or mouth.

PREGNANCY

❧

If there is a history of miscarriage it is advisable not to use essential oils.

It is also not advisable to use even the low toxicity (safe) oils for long periods of time during any pregnancy.

Assuming everything is normal aromatherapy treatments can be very beneficial.

During the first three months when the foetus is very vulnerable, oils such as Geranium, Ginger, Grapefruit, Alpine Lavender, Mandarin and Roman Camomile may be used. Do not use any other oil.

Four months onwards the oil range may be extended to include Cypress, Fennel, Jasmine, Peppermint, Rose and Rosewood. Massage should be gentle, preferably on the upper back, neck and shoulders. Compresses and vaporizers are an alternative. The dilution should be 20 mls of carrier oil, with 5 drops of a chosen essential oil.

Morning sickness. This may be helped by inhaling Ginger or Peppermint.

Post Natal Depression may be helped by a compress or vaporizer, by applying 2 drops of Bergamot, Geranium, Alpine Lavender, Neroli, Rose or Rosewood.

Stretch Marks. From the end of the fifth month these may be helped by a gentle massage. Take 20 mls Sweet Almond oil and 5 mls Wheatgerm oil, add 2 drops of Alpine Lavender, 2 drops Mandarin and 2 drops Neroli. Gently massage the abdomen in a clockwise direction until all the oil has been absorbed. This can be applied night and morning, right up to the time of birth.

Varicose Veins. These may be helped by a compress with Cypress oil.

THE ELDERLY

Age tends to come at different speeds. Some people can be quite feeble and inactive at sixty-five, whilst others are bursting with energy at ninety.

There is less resistance to disease, a slower recovery rate, and they can often be on intensive medication.

The heart, liver, lungs and kidneys are very rarely functioning to full extent. Excretion is often affected, so they could be at risk of oil toxicity, if used long term.

BONE AND MUSCLE DEGENERATION
Often causes pain, sometimes quite severely. Treatments should therefore be less often. Suggested time 20 minutes, once a week.

COMPRESSES, INHALATIONS, HAND AND FOOT BATHS
All are very useful. Add 2-3 drops of essential oil for a 20 minute treatment.

LOCALIZED MASSAGE
Can be very helpful. Take 20 mls carrier oil and add 5-6 drops of a chosen essential oil.

A rich carrier oil such as Avocado, Evening Primrose or Jojoba should be chosen for the frail dry skin and bony areas. The essential oil should be a safe cosseting oil, such as Alpine Lavender, Frankincense, Neroli, Rose or Sandalwood Mysore.

DEPRESSION AND LOW SELF-ESTEEM

This may be helped by a gentle massage, or inhaling the vapours of the oils of Bergamot, Geranium, Jasmine, Rose or Sandalwood Mysore.

DIGESTIVE PROBLEMS

These can be real problems for the aged and are often relieved by adding 1-2 drops of Black Pepper, Ginger, Peppermint, Patchouli or Rosemary on a compress and placed on the stomach area. Alternatively, inhale the vapours.

FADING MEMORY

This may be helped by a gentle massage of the shoulders, hands or feet, using the stimulating oils of Alpine Lavender, Basil, Bergamot or Rosemary. Inhaling the vapours is also an alternative.

INSOMNIA

Very helpful by vaporizing 1-2 drops of the soothing oils of Alpine Lavender, Camomile, Mandarin, Neroli, Petitgrain. Place in bedroom one hour before retiring.

THE TERMINALLY ILL

❧

This condition should not be treated unless the consultant or GP consents.

Until quite recently, cancer was something that people died from. It now appears that it is an illness people can learn to live with and many years of life can follow the diagnosis.

By the use of aromatherapy oils we can create a caring environment, thus enhancing the quality of life of the patient.

In nearly all cases massage should not be used as the patient's immune system would be under extreme stress from chemotherapy, drugs, radiotherapy and surgery, or perhaps a combination of all. Also the patient is vulnerable to infections.

Inhalations and room vaporizers would be helpful. Select the oils of Alpine Lavender, Eucalyptus or Tea Tree which will boost the immune system. 2 drops only should be used.

In some cases, a gentle hand or foot massage may be beneficial using a rich carrier oil only.

Areas subject to radiotherapy must not be treated and no essential oil used during chemotherapy, due to the liver working overtime and severe nausea being a problem.

As the emotional system is also under extreme pressure, essential oils can be vaporized to support the patient for the physical and mental wellbeing they can create as follows:

EMOTIONAL BALANCER	Geranium
BODY AND MIND UNWINDERS	Frankincense, Jasmine, Mandarin, Rose, Rosewood, Sandalwood Mysore, Vetivert
GENERAL TONICS	Alpine Lavender, Mandarin
SPIRIT LIFTERS	Bergamot, Patchouli, Petitgrain, Ylang-Ylang extra
STRESS RELIEVERS	Clary Sage, Neroli

RECIPES

All the following recipes have all been thoroughly tried and tested by myself and my clients over the last twenty-five years.

BATHS

ACHES/PAINS (General)	5-6 drops Camomile or 3 drops Lavender 3 drops Eucalyptus
COMFORTING	5 drops Patchouli
FLUID RETENTION	5-6 drops Juniperberry
FORTIFYING (Boosts Immune System)	2 drops Tea Tree 2 drops Lavender 1 drop Juniperberry
HARMONIZING/BALANCING	5 drops Lavender 2 drops Geranium
HIGH BLOOD PRESSURE	6-8 drops Alpine Lavender (due to stress)
HANGOVER	2 drops Fennel 4 drops Juniperberry 2 drops Rosemary

INSOMNIA/DEPRESSION

5-6 drops Rose
OR
5-6 drops Neroli
OR
3 drops Alpine Lavender
3 drops Mandarin
OR
3 drops Alpine Lavender
1 drop Camomile
2 drops Petitgrain

JOINT PAIN

4 drops Red Thyme
2 drops Cedarwood

NERVOUS FATIGUE

4 drops Marjoram
2 drops Orange
OR
2 drops Basil
4 drops Geranium

PICK-ME-UP

5-6 drops Rosewood
OR
4 drops Rosewood
2 drops Ylang-Ylang extra
OR
2 drops Orange
2 drops Rose

RELAXING

5-6 drops Neroli (ultra, ultra)
OR
2 drops Alpine Lavender
2 drops Patchouli
2 drops Rose

OR
4 drops Sandalwood Mysore
2 drops Ylang-Ylang extra
OR
4 drops Lavender
2 drops Ylang-Ylang extra

REVITALIZING (for a special date)

4 drops Rosewood
2 drops Bergamot
OR
2 drops Neroli
2 drops Rose
2 drops Sandalwood Mysore

SENSUAL

2 drops Sandalwood Mysore
2 drops Ylang-Ylang extra
1 drop Jasmine
OR
2 drops Rose
2 drops Sandalwood Mysore
1 drop Clary Sage
OR
1 drop Bergamot
1 drop Jasmine or Rose
3 drops Sandalwood Mysore

STIMULATING (early morning)

5-6 drops Rosemary
OR
3 drops Bergamot
3 drops Rosemary
OR
3 drops Juniperberry
1 drop Peppermint
2 drops Rosemary

N.B. Do not put more than 10 drops in a bath in 24 hours

INHALATIONS

CATARRH, CHEST INFECTIONS:
2-3 drops Benzoin into a bowl of hot water. Inhale deeply through the nose. This balsamic resin is soothing and uplifting. Repeat as necessary.

COLDS, CATARRH, HAYFEVER, MIGRAINE, LOSS OF SMELL, SINUS CONGESTION:
3-4 drops Basil into bowl of hot water. Inhale for approximately 5 minutes up to three times per day until condition improves.

BRONCHITIS, CATARRH, COUGHS, COLDS, INFLUENZA, VIRAL INFECTIONS:
3-4 drops Eucalyptus in a bowl of hot water. Inhale for 5-6 minutes. Use as necessary.

HEADACHES, COLDS, COUGHS, INFLUENZA, MIGRAINE, FACIAL NEURALGIA:
3 drops Camomile in a bowl of hot water. Inhale for 5-6 minutes. Repeat when necessary.

RESPIRATORY CONGESTION, CATARRH DISCHARGE, EXCELLENT FOR ALL MUCOUS CONDITIONS:
3-4 drops Frankincense in a bowl of hot water. Inhale deeply through the nose for 6-8 minutes. Repeat up to three times a day until condition improves. Once the catarrh begins to liquefy the oil can be changed to Basil. Repeat as necessary.

ASTHMA, DECONGESTANT, HEADACHES, INFLUENZA, MIGRAINE, NAUSEA:
3-4 drops French Lavender OR 2-3 drops Peppermint in a bowl of hot water. Use as necessary.

CHEST COMPLAINTS, LUNG INFECTIONS, SORE THROATS, TONSILLITIS:
5 drops Sandalwood Mysore in a bowl of hot water. Inhale for approximately 7-8 minutes to allow the soothing vapours to penetrate. Use up to three times per day.

ASTHMA, BRONCHITIS, CATARRH, CHEST, EAR, NOSE AND THROAT INFECTIONS, COUGHS, COLDS, RESPIRATORY CONGESTION, SINUSITIS, WHOOPING COUGH, BOOSTS THE IMMUNE SYSTEM:
4 drops Tea Tree in a bowl of hot water. Inhale deeply for 5-6 minutes. Repeat if necessary.

CONGESTED HEAD COLDS:
1 drop Basil, 3 drops Eucalyptus, 1 drop Peppermint in a bowl of hot water. Inhale for 5-6 minutes. Use as necessary.

INFLUENZA:
1 drop Black Pepper, 1 drop Camphor, 3 drops Eucalyptus in a bowl of hot water. Inhale for 5-6 minutes. Use as necessary.

MASSAGE

The following massage recipes are for blends of essential oils mixed in 20 mls of carrier oil. I find this amount just right for a complete body massage without being wasteful.

ACHES/PAINS (General)

6 drops Camomile or
4 drops Rosemary
(Also a tonic for the liver)
OR

6 drops Lavender
3 drops Ginger
1 drop Melisa

~

COMFORTING/COSSETING

6 drops Lavender
2 drops Rose
2 drops Rosewood
OR
3 drops Bergamot
4 drops Clary Sage
3 drops Ylang-Ylang extra

~

DE-STRESSING

5 drops Camomile
3 drops Rose
2 drops Vetivert
OR
5 drops Bergamot
3 drops Frankincense
2 drops Jasmine
OR
6 drops Lavender
2 drops Rose
2 drops Neroli

~

DEPRESSION, FRIGIDITY, INSOMNIA

10 drops Rose Otto or
Absolute
Excellent for full body
massage, facial massage and
broken capillaries.

~

GENERAL FATIGUE, IRRITABILITY

10 drops Clary Sage
Very good all round panacea
for full body, or localized
massage

INFLUENZA, VIRAL INFECTIONS

2 drops Eucalyptus
6 drops Lavender
2 drops Pine
Massage chest and back until
warmth is felt

INVIGORATING

1 drop Juniperberry
2 drops Lemon
7 drops Rosemary
OR
1 drop Geranium
3 drops Orange
6 drops Rosewood

NERVOUS DEPRESSION

2 drops Bergamot
5 drops Rose
3 drops Sandalwood Mysore
OR
5 drops Neroli add to 10 mls
carrier oil. Massage clock-
wise over the solar plexus for
15-20 minutes, preferably at
bedtime

NERVOUS INSOMNIA

7 drops Basil
3 drops Marjoram
Apply to full body or neck
and shoulders

RELAXING/SOOTHING

2 drops Clary Sage
7 drops Lavender
1 drop Rose
OR
3 drops Camomile
6 drops Lavender
1 drop Marjoram

SENSUAL

2 drops Neroli
6 drops Sandalwood Mysore
2 drops Ylang-Ylang extra
OR
1 drop Jasmine
6 drops Sandalwood Mysore
3 drops Ylang-Ylang extra
OR
1 drop Clary Sage
2 drops Geranium
7 drops Ylang-Ylang extra
OR
1 drop Jasmine
6 drops Rosewood
3 drops Ylang-Ylang extra

STIMULATING, TONIC

3 drops Cedarwood
5 drops Lavender
2 drops Rosemary

ROOM METHODS

The following oils are anti-bacterial and anti-viral; also depression fighters. All are excellent for clearing the atmosphere, bringing freshness and clarity to any occasion, or any crowded room.

Choose a method to create a mood suitable for a specific occasion by means of an oil burner, light bulbs, radiators, aroma-stones or aromastream vaporizers.

Add 2,3 or 4 drops to suit your taste.

AFTERNOON TEA/LADIES SEWING CIRCLE	Geranium
BARBECUE/DISCO	Bergamot or Rosewood
CELEBRATORY DINNER PARTY	Cinnamon or Sandalwood
CHILDREN'S PARTIES	Mandarin or Orange
ENGAGEMENT PARTY/ ST. VALENTINE'S DAY	Geranium, Jasmine, Rose or Ylang-Ylang extra
TEENAGER'S SPECIAL BIRTHDAY	Rose
CHRISTMAS EVE through to NEW YEAR'S DAY	Cedarwood, Cinnamon Frankincense, Mandarin or Petitgrain

Any Occasion:

ATMOSPHERE CLEANSERS e.g. Tobacco smoke, airborne diseases	Bergamot, Lemon, Lemongrass, Melisa and Rosewood
AIDS SLEEP/REDUCES ANXIETY	Alpine Lavender
BEDROOM FRAGRANCES	Jasmine, Patchouli, Rose, Sandalwood Mysore, Ylang-Ylang extra
CONFIDENCE BUILDER	Jasmine

CRISIS SOOTHER	Basil
DEPRESSION LIFTERS	Clary Sage or Ylang-Ylang extra
IMMUNE SYSTEM BOOSTERS	Bergamot, Lavender, Lemon-grass, Rosewood, Sandalwood Mysore, Tea Tree
STIMULATING	Peppermint
UNWIND AFTER A STRESSFUL DAY	Geranium, Lavender, Neroli Rosewood

No doubt you will think of other occasions, or situations, in which to use the special powers of the essential oils, to make **THAT** moment extra special. After a little experience, you will know the right combinations to blend a wonderful aroma, to create the **MOOD** you require.

Always remember that each oil has got its own rather unique personality, just like each one of your friends.

MISCELLANEOUS FORMULAE

AROMATHERAPY FOR MEN

CLARY SAGE	all round panacea
CYPRESS	invigorating
FRANKINCENSE	nervous tension, aid to meditation and spiritual development
GERANIUM	uplifting, balancer and harmonizer
LAVENDER	balances mind and body; relaxing
LEMON	detoxifying, refreshing
ROSEMARY	improves memory, aids concentration
ROSEWOOD	stabilizing, rejuvenating
SANDALWOOD	boosts the immune system, insomnia, and relaxation

These oils can be used for baths, massage and vaporizing.

ACHING FEET/AFTER SHOPPING, WALKING OR SICK HEADACHE

Revive in a footbath of warm water, adding 3 drops Lavender, 1 drop Peppermint, 2 drops Rosemary for 10-15 minutes.

AWAY FROM HOME/OVERNIGHT OR HOLIDAYS

Pack the oils of Bergamot, Lavender or Rosewood. Sprinkle a few drops over the carpets in the bathroom and bedroom to freshen and protect against airborne bacteria and stale tobacco odours.

BASIL

A very popular herb to have growing in the kitchen garden close to the kitchen door, as it is an excellent insect repellent, including mosquitoes.

BAY

Bay trees are also popular to have at the front door, as Bay has proved itself over the years. It is a strong insect repellent.

BEAT THE AFTER LUNCH SLUMP

For an instant energy lift put 1-2 drops of Peppermint Oil onto a tissue and inhale. The aroma will quickly awaken your senses to help you feel renewed. It is easy, fast and feels great.

BURNS

For small burns apply 1-2 drops of neat Lavender oil immediately. It will feel better very quickly. Re-apply if necessary. For large burns, to a large bowl of cold water add 12 drops of Lavender oil and immerse the affected part for 15-20 minutes. Lavender neat, or in water, will reduce the pain and heat, calm the patient and aid rapid healing in 3-5 days, without a scar. Second degree burns in 5-7 days.

CEDARWOOD, ROSEWOOD, SANDALWOOD OR VETIVERT

All are excellent as moth repellents. Place 2-3 drops of your chosen oil on blotting paper and put into your drawers and wardrobes. They are a wonderful replacement for moth balls.

CHICKEN POX

To cool the itching spots, add 1 drop of Peppermint oil to 5 pints of water. Apply to spots with a cotton wool bud, as necessary. Continue until spots start to dry.

CIRCULATORY PROBLEMS

Broken facial capillaries – mix 10mls carrier oil with 3 drops Cypress oil. Apply with a gentle massage to the area twice daily.

Haemorrhoids – put 2-3 drops Cypress oil in bidet, or bowl of warm water, sit in for 10-15 minutes, then blot dry.

Varicose Veins – mix 10mls carrier oil with 3 drops Cypress oil and gently massage up the legs once a day.

EARACHE

Put 1 drop Lavender oil on cotton wool, gently place in ear. The warm healing vapours will help relieve the pain.

EXHAUSTION, FAINTING, FRIGHT AND SHOCK

Use the powerful oils of Basil, Peppermint or Rosemary. Put 1-2 drops on a tissue and pass to and fro under the nose.

FUNGAL INFECTION OF THE NAILS

Apply 1 drop of neat Tea Tree onto the nail twice each day. Take care not to get the oil onto the surrounding skin. Continue application until new nail grows up.

HAEMATOSIS

Prepare a compress to dissolve the bruise by adding 2-3 drops Geranium oil. It makes the blood more fluid, and has a general effect on circulation.

HAIR LOSS

Mix 20mls Jojoba oil with 10 drops Rosemary oil, or 5 drops Rosemary and 5 drops Lavender. Apply daily. Massage scalp for 10-15 minutes, or until the scalp feels quite warm. Continue treatment until new hair starts to appear.

HRT – LITTLE HELPER
Place a burner or vaporizer in the bedroom. Add 1-2 drops of Geranium, Camomile or Rose. Leave for approximately 1 hour before retiring.

HAVING AN 'OFF DAY'
Put 1 drop of Clary Sage oil onto a tissue and inhale, or vaporize 2-3 drops for its euphoric effect.

HEALING, SOOTHING
Irritated, dry, cracked skin can be helped with 20mls. carrier oil and 10 drops Benzoin oil. Massage gently. Leave on overnight. The stimulating resin will strengthen the skin tissue.

INFECTED FACIAL SPOTS
Using a cotton wool bud, apply neat Tea Tree three times per day. When the pus has cleared, apply neat Lavender in the same way. This will prevent scarring.

JET LAG
Often described as chronic tiredness, constipation, insomnia, swollen ankles, feet and legs, with perhaps confusion and depression. Possibly more acute in some people than in others. These feelings can last up to 3-5 days, all due to eating more frequently, travelling at high speeds and sitting still for eight hours or more. On reaching destination bathe, if possible with 6 drops Lavender oil, for a relaxed sleep. If you have a business meeting to attend bathe with 5-6 drops of Rosemary oil, to freshen and energize, and to see you through the day. These baths can be used night and morning, until the body has adjusted. Avoid alcohol, drink plenty of still mineral water and only eat when hungry. For that uplifting feeling, place 2 drops Clary Sage on a tissue and inhale as necessary.

LAVENDER

It is a well-known fact that most Spanish men use Lavender toiletries to keep insects and particularly mosquitoes at bay. In September 1998, German scientists found that mosquitoes hated the scent of Lavender, Peppermint and Tomato plants, and all are natural repellents.

PERFUME FOR DRAWERS

Excellent for the lingerie drawer. 2-3 drops on blotting paper of either Geranium, Patchouli, Rose or Ylang-Ylang.

SHINGLES

Bathe the affected part with Bergamot, Geranium or Peppermint. To 6-7 pints of cold water, add 2 drops of your chosen oil. Apply as necessary.

THROAT PROBLEMS

Whether it be loss of voice, sore throat, or tonsillitis, Sandalwood will take care of it. Mix 20mls. carrier oil with 10 drops of essential oil. Massage morning and night under ears and all around front of neck, down on to chest.

TORTICOLLIS OR WRY-NECK

This condition is on a contraction of one or more of the cervical muscles on one side only, resulting in an abnormal position of the head. Mix 20mls. carrier oil with 10 drops Clary Sage oil and massage daily, if possible. If only weekly treatments are given, it can take 4-6 months for healing to take place.

TRAVEL OR MOTION SICKNESS

When driving, flying or sailing, always take with you Lavender and Peppermint oils. Lavender soothes the psyche; Peppermint calms the stomach. Adults – 2-3 drops on a tissue, inhale as necessary. Children – 1 drop on a tissue. Adults only – in severe cases mix 20mls. carrier oil, add 10 drops Ginger oil, and massage the stomach area in a clock-wise direction, night and morning until the nausea has passed. If oil not available, chew Crystallised Ginger to help the sickness. It works every time.

To conclude, I have been using Aromatherapy for over twenty-five years, and it is one of the most rewarding treatments for both my clients and myself. It is a therapy which has proved itself over thousands of years to be one of the finest known to Mankind. I have had enormous pleasure and satisfaction in my work, which I hope continues for many more years. The more I work with the oils, and see the results, I feel very humble.

After all the plants give us life and we, in the end, give plants life.

INDEX